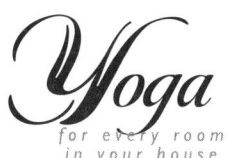

Yoga
for every room
in your house

Yoga

for every room in your house

Jinjer Stanton

Great Bear Press • Minneapolis

© 2010 Jinjer Stanton. All rights reserved.

Published by
Great Bear Press, Minneapolis, Minnesota
www.greatbearpress.net
Photographs by Jinjer Stanton

Book design by Dorie McClelland, Spring Book Design,
www.springbookdesign.com

ISBN: 978-0-578-04418-7

Dedicated to Aunt Viv and Uncle Ken
who believed in me more than I believed in myself.

Yoga

Introduction *xiii*

basics
Breathing *2*
To Train Yourself to Breathe Properly *4*
Integrating Breath and Movement *6*
Breath and Stress *8*
Moving Mindfully *9*
Symmetry *10*
The Power of the Mind *11*

in the bedroom
Can You Stand It? *14*
Bear Hug *14*
Carnival Ride *16*
Bear Hug and Carnival Ride *18*
Neck Stretches *20*
Shoulder Circles *22*
Chicken Arms *24*
Side Bend *26*
Forward Bend *28*
Backbend *30*

Twisting, Turning . . . *32*
Flat on Your Back *34*
Hamstring Stretch *35*
Toe-Grabbing Fun *38*
Cross Your Legs *40*
Restorative Pose *42*
Legs Up the Wall *44*
Face Massage—Sweet Dreams *46*
If All Else Fails, Meditate *48*

in the bathroom

Cow Face Pose *50*
Cat on the Tub *52*
Bathing the Kids Squat *54*
The Neti Pot *56*
Twisting, Turning . . . Reprise *58*

in the kitchen

Mountain Pose and Meditation *62*
Standing Hamstring Stretch *64*
Palm Tree *66*
Pine Tree *68*
Kitchen Warrior I *70*
Kitchen Warrior II *72*
Supported Forward Bend *74*
Backbend *76*
Plank at the Counter, Table, or Chair Seat *78*

Dog in a Chair   *80*
Knee Circles   *82*
Do You Have a Dining Room?   *84*

in the living room
Fingers, Hands and Wrists   *86*
Toes and Feet   *90*
Scaring the Cat   *94*
Lion Pose   *96*

in the office
Angel Rescue Mission   *100*
Reversing Gravity: The Shoulder Stand   *102*
The Shoulder Stand Made Easy   *104*
Legs in Chair Pose   *106*
Torso Flip   *108*
Repeating the Good Stuff   *110*
Supported Forward Bend . . . Revisited   *110*
Supported Backbend . . . Revisited   *112*
Dog in a Chair . . . Revisited   *114*
Cow Face Pose . . . Revisited   *116*
Fingers, Hands and Wrists . . . Revisited   *118*
Twisting, Turning . . . Revisited   *120*
Seated Forward Bend . . . Revisited   *122*
Backbend   *124*

Out of India
- You Are a Yogi   *127*
- Hindu/Scriptural History   *129*
- Yoga's Nitty Gritty   *132*
- Other Useful Things to Know About   *144*
- A Sampling of Yoga Styles   *147*
- Resources   *150*

Acknowledgments   *159*

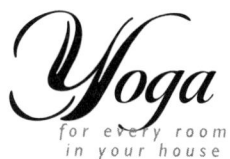

Yoga
for every room in your house

Introduction

It always feels I'm like putting my body back together when I do yoga, especially when I've let it slide for a while. And it's easy to let it slide when there's no designated space for yoga. Especially when it's winter and the wind is howling out of the north, the car's broken down and class is ten blocks away or across town.

For a short time I lived with a dancer who kept the living room free of furniture so she could practice. That was great because whenever I felt like doing a little yoga there was space clear for a complete workout. However, at no other time in my life has there been clear space for yoga in my home. I'm way too lazy to move furniture to make room, then move the furniture back. Because of that, I have generally just not done yoga unless I was taking a class or teaching one.

Yet, over time, I've found that there are times when I absolutely *had* to do yoga in order to get work done, stay healthy or fall asleep at night. Since necessity is the mother of invention, I modified some poses and simply transferred others to situations they aren't normally used in. Perhaps the most radical of these is the shoulder stand I did once in a deserted meeting room at work, wearing a skirt and nylons. It was a day when I was on deadline and I had a bad head cold that kept me from thinking clearly. A couple of minutes with my legs straight up in the air made a world of difference in my ability to do my job. Every time I think of that day I give up a prayer of thanksgiving that no one walked in while I was upside down!

Some of these exercises were developed for a student with one leg.

This collection of poses (asanas, exercises) is designed to be within the capabilities of most people and still provide many of the benefits of traditional poses.

This book is not intended to replace a regular yoga class or regular yoga practice (though if the choice is these exercises or no yoga at all, do these exercises). It is intended to supplement those things when circumstances are not friendly to doing yoga in the traditional way. It is also intended to encourage a yoga practice full of joy and pleasure as well as ensuring you experience the wonderful benefits to health and well-being documented from ancient times. It may be that people for whom yoga has seemed inaccessible (for whatever reason) may be inspired by some of these ideas.

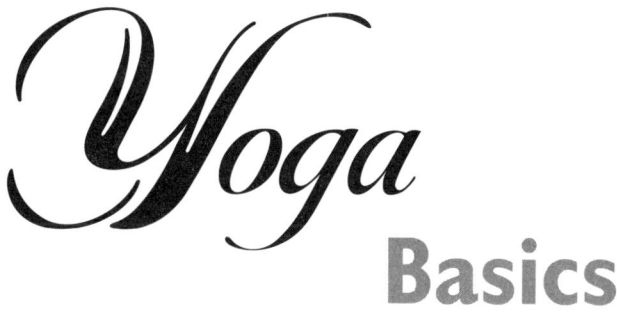
Yoga Basics

These principles are the bedrock of a healthy yoga practice. Keep them in mind whenever you practice yoga whether in class or on your own. They will serve you well.

Yoga Basics

Breathing

We all know how to breathe—sort of. Our bodies just do it and very little consciousness is involved in the process unless something happens that makes breathing difficult. Singers and musicians who play various horns and flutes are a bit more conscious. They've had to learn to control their breathing in order to get the best from their instruments and voices.

Our lungs are smaller at the top and larger toward the bottom, and when they are full they can hold around eight quarts of air. However, most of us use nowhere near our full lung capacity. Many exchange as little as two quarts of air in a given breath. Yoga practice helps us regain our optimal lung capacity.

All by itself healthy breathing has a powerful impact on our lives in terms of our general health and well-being—not to mention our mental and spiritual functioning and development. Healthy breathing increases life expectancy and helps alleviate medical conditions like asthma, poor digestion, insomnia, low energy, high blood pressure, stress, panic attacks, heart disease, and more. Healthy breathing also helps us metabolize food more effectively. That's why I encourage proper breathing and integration of breath in the practice of yoga.

We can trick ourselves into breathing properly by lying on our bellies and resting our foreheads on our arms. Try this to see how it feels. Notice how your belly expands and lifts you upwards as you inhale then lowers you back down as you exhale.

Yoga Basics

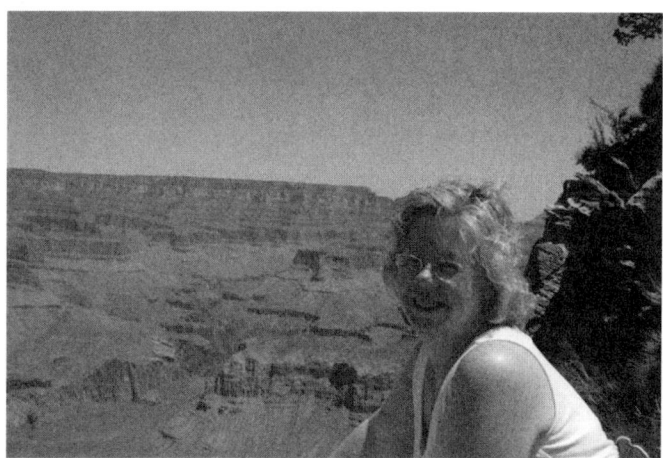

Sue breathing deep at high altitude

Recently, a student (Sue Olson) who has only been studying with me a few months went on a mountain vacation with her husband (who is not practicing yoga). Because of her increased lung capacity from her yoga practice she was comfortable and vigorous at the highest altitudes while her husband was panting and forced to take frequent breaks!

Yoga Basics

To Train Yourself to Breathe Properly

1. Stand or sit upright with your spine straight. If you have developed a habitual slouch, consciously pull your shoulder blades together and lift your chest.

2. Inhale slowly and deeply while consciously expanding your belly until it is round and tight.

3. Continue to inhale while filling your chest until it is full and tight. You can even tilt your head back a little to make sure every bit of lung space is full. You may feel slight discomfort from being so full of air if it's been a while since your lungs were really full.

4. Begin exhaling slowly from top to bottom so that your chest empties first, then your abdomen.

5. When you think your lungs are empty, continue to exhale while rounding your shoulders and back to squeeze out any stale air still hiding in the corners. Now, you don't need to do this step for every breath you take, but it's a good idea to empty the lungs completely at least once a day.

6. Repeat from Step 1 several times.

If you get light-headed, stop. Try again tomorrow, and the next day and the next. Little by little you'll increase your ability to breathe well and deeply and will become healthier and healthier. Add side bends to your practice. This will stretch the muscles between your ribs and help you cultivate greater lung capacity (*see* in the Bedroom *or* in the Living Room *for how to do sidebends*).

Yoga Basics

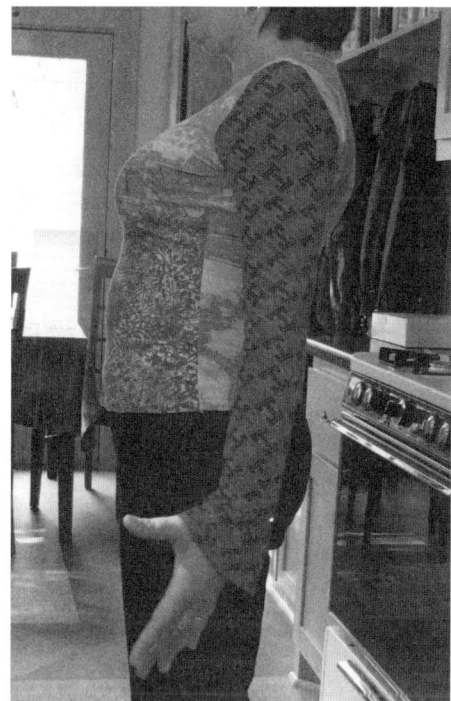

Inhale

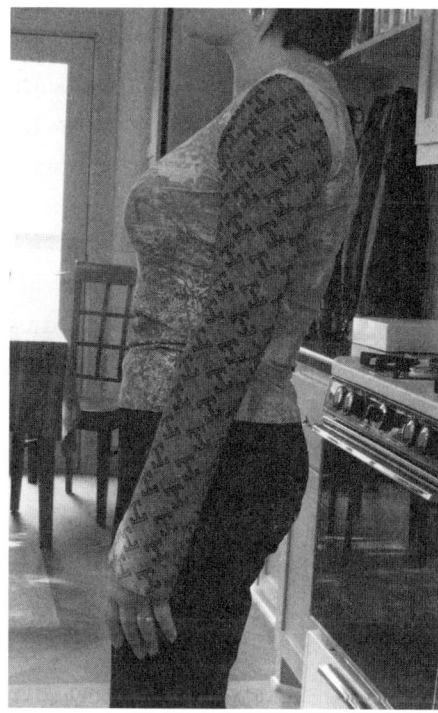

Exhale

Yoga Basics

Integrating Breath and Movement

Breath can help us in our yoga practice if we learn to coordinate our breathing with the exercises (called asanas, poses, or postures). The rule of thumb is this: Inhale when the chest is opening and exhale as it's being compressed.

What that means is, if our arms are up or out to the side, if we are bending backwards or stretching upwards, the chest is opening and we should be inhaling. If our arms are in front or we are bending forward, the chest is being compressed and we should exhale.

Yoga Basics

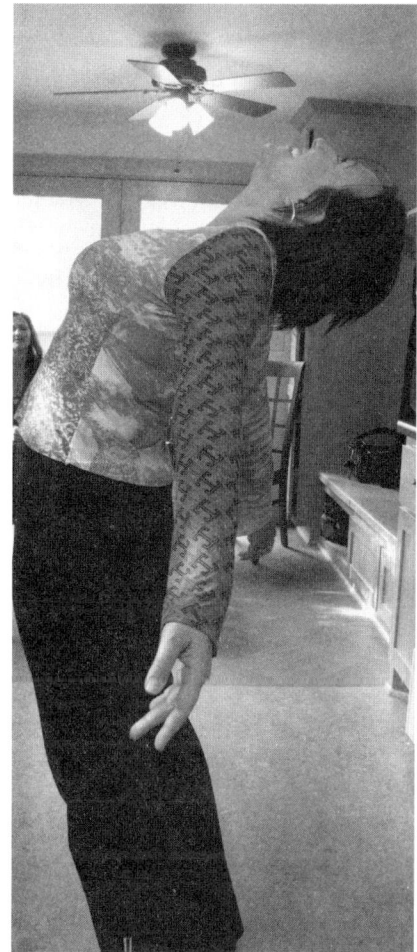

Inhale

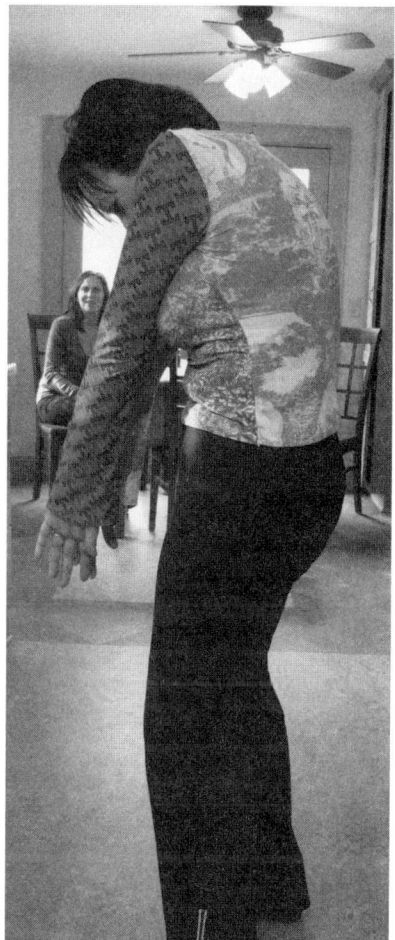

Exhale

Yoga Basics

Breath and Stress

One excellent place to use our increased awareness of our breath is when we are under stress.

Stress causes us to tense up and decreases the volume of air we inhale, which causes more stress, which causes us to tense up even more, which causes us to breathe yet more shallowly, which . . .

. . . Makes me tense just thinking about it. If we can bring our attention to our breath when we are under stress and consciously breathe more deeply, we handle the stress much better and are less likely to get some of the diseases associated with stress.

Yoga Basics

Moving Mindfully

I have just two rules for my yoga classes:

1. **Don't compare yourself to others!** If you can't do all of the poses as easily as others seem to but you do the best you are capable of, you still receive the benefits. Every body is different. You can probably do something else easily that others have trouble with. Also, it is inevitable that you will improve over time. Be gentle with yourself.

2. **Pay attention to your own body and emotions.** If something seems scary, don't do it. If something is painful, either back off until it doesn't hurt anymore or don't do it at all. This is particularly important if you are practicing without a teacher. Even if you are practicing with a teacher, that teacher may not know what's going on with you. Every body is different. Respect yours and trust your own experience.

Also, paying attention through all the exercises increases the benefit you get from them and increases your awareness of what's going on with your body at other times.

Yoga Basics

Symmetry

A simple yogic rule is: If you bend forward, make sure you bend back to balance it. If you do something on the right side, be sure to do it on the left as well. Consistency with this will gradually bring your body into balance.

Even if you are missing an arm or leg, you can apply this rule energetically through visualization. Do as much as you can and imagine the rest. Remember, the physical limb may be missing, but energetically it's still there—that's what a ghost limb is. Your whole body will thank you if you put in this effort.

Yoga Basics

The Power of the Mind

Those of us who happen to still own a full complement of limbs can also use imagination in aid of our yoga practice. Any time a pose seems scary or your body just isn't ready to attempt it don't just sit there feeling rotten. Instead, close your eyes, go inside and imagine the doing of it, giving full attention to each movement, each sensation. All things we once could not do, we come to be able to do by way of imagination.

We know this works anecdotally by way of sports figures. We hear an Olympic champion say in an interview, "Just this morning I ran through my routine [or the course, or my dive, etc.] in my mind and it was perfect. It went exactly the same way during competition." When the favorite who came in fourth is interviewed the conversation goes something like this:

Interviewer: "So, what went wrong out there today?"

Athlete: "I dunno. When I tried to picture my race [or routine, or . . .] I just couldn't see myself winning!"

I've heard of a couple of studies that demonstrate the power of imagination in physical prowess. In the Wikipedia article on creative visualization it says:

"Just before the 1980 Olympics, the Russian coaches and scientists did tests with the athletes comparing mental training and physical training methods.

"Russian scientists compared four groups of Olympic athletes in terms of their training schedules:

"Group 1: 100% physical training;

"Group 2: 75% physical training with 25% mental training;

"Group 3: 50% physical training with 50% mental training;

Yoga Basics

"Group 4: 25% physical training with 75% mental training.

"Group 4, with 75% of their time devoted to mental training, performed the best. 'The Soviets had discovered that mental images can act as a prelude to muscular impulses.'"

—*Karate of Okinawa*, Robert Scaglione and William Cummins

The second study is said to have been conducted by Dr. Blaslotto, a basketball coach at the University of Chicago. He had his players practice free-throws together for an hour. Then he divided the players into three groups. The first group was told to not even think of basketball for a month. The second group practiced free-throws for an hour every day. The third group spent an hour a day visualizing throwing perfect free-throws.

When the players were evaluated at the end of the month, the first group had not improved at all. The second group had improved by 24%. The third group improved by 23%!

Finally, a woman I knew once suffered an injury that made it impossible for her to get up out of bed because the pain in her back was so bad. Doctors told her there was a good chance she would never walk again. Daily she spent time imagining rolling over, dangling her legs off the edge of the bed, and standing up.

At first, she just couldn't make it happen even in the privacy of her own mind. But over time she got better at imagining it. Finally, she did it physically.

Just a little something to remember when you are confronted by a challenge a little larger than you think you can handle.

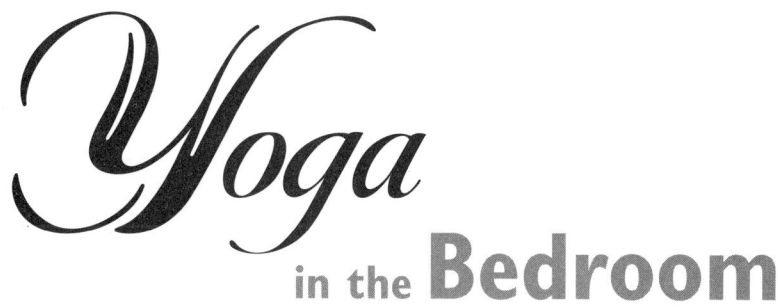

Yoga in the Bedroom

You can use yoga at the edge of your bed to help you get to sleep (if you suffer from insomnia) or to help you get out of bed in the morning (if you wake up stiff).

If your bed is too tall for you to feel stable with your legs hanging over the edge, just throw on a robe and move to a chair or a couch for these poses.

in the Bedroom

Can You Stand It?

Now, if you can manage to do these first two warm-ups standing you'll get more benefit from them because of the increased range of motion. Also, your chances of sending lamp, clock or reading material flying across the room diminish sharply.

Usually, if I'm tossing and turning I decide at some point that a trip to the bathroom will help. I time these exercises for when I'm coming back.

Bear Hug

Stand with your feet shoulder width apart in an area where you can swing your arms freely without crashing into anything. Inhale as you throw your arms wide as though you are about to hug someone very dear to you. As you exhale, throw your arms around yourself in a big bear hug that squeezes the breath out of you.

Repeat this several times making sure that you are inhaling as your arms fly open and exhaling as they wrap around you again. Alternate which arm comes out on top during the hug portion of the movement.

The bear hug helps loosen tight shoulders, replace stale air with fresh and promotes self-esteem. To increase this last benefit you can repeat to yourself, "I love you," and "You done good."

in the Bedroom

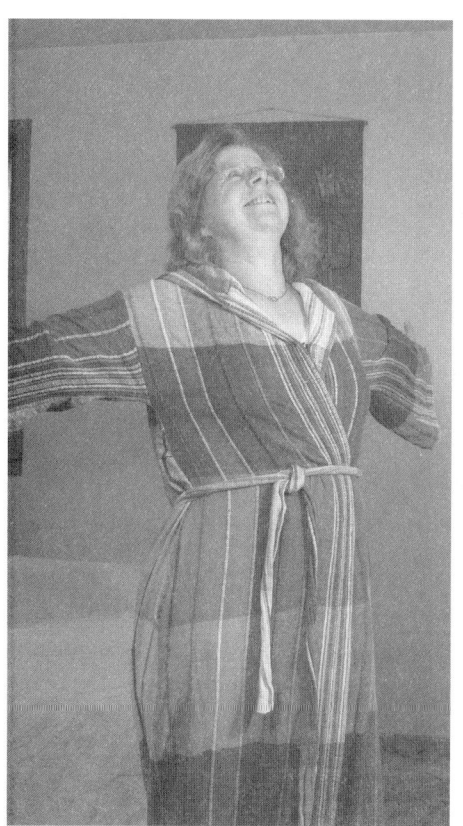
Inhale

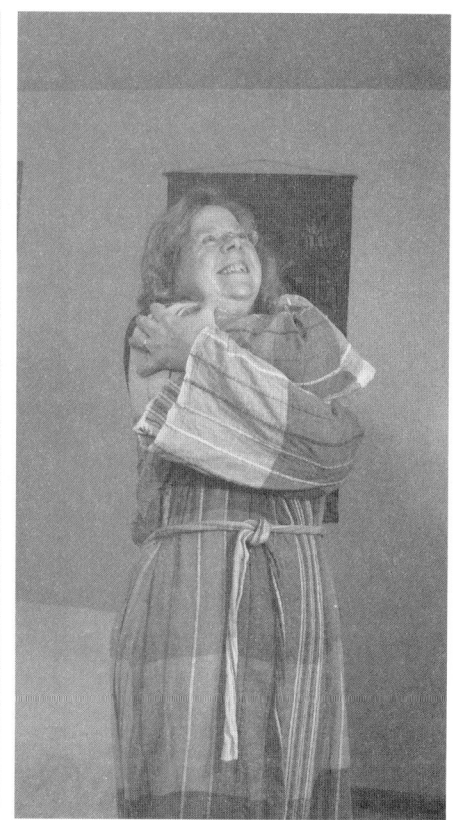
Exhale

in the **Bedroom**

Carnival Ride

I love this one. You start out in the same position as the bear hug only now you gently rotate your upper body back and forth around your waist letting your arms fly free. Turn your head to follow the arm that's flying back at any given point.

This exercise, all by itself, can go a long way toward massaging away any tension in your back while increasing flexibility. It's also very pleasant. It reminds me of that amusement park ride where swings are suspended from a great wheel and as the wheel rotates the swings begin to gently fly outward from the center due to centrifugal force.

in the Bedroom

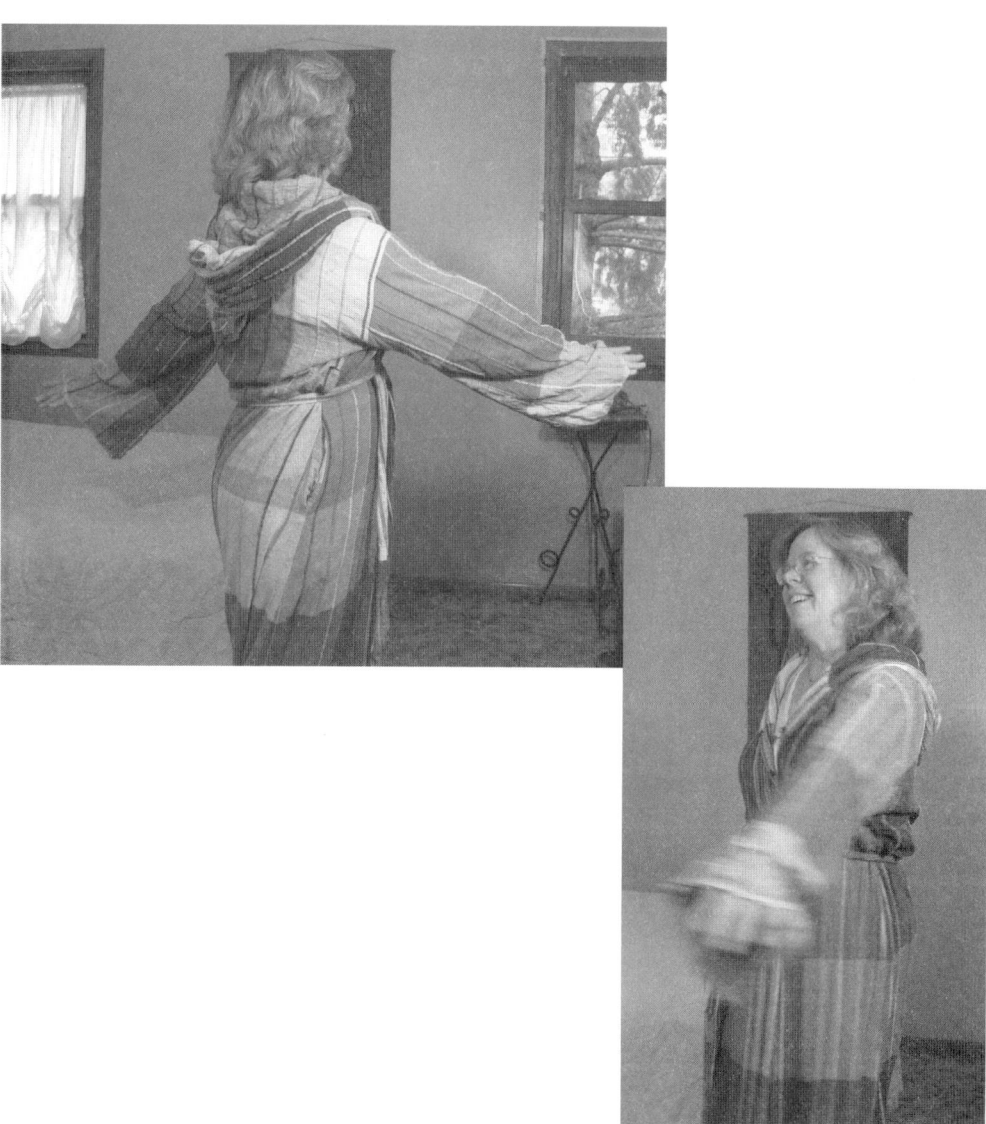

in the Bedroom

*Watch Out for Flying Lamps or,
What to Do if You **Can't** Stand It*

Bear Hug and Carnival Ride

You can do these sitting down at the edge of your bed. They're just not quite as effective and there are those lamps and lovers' faces to watch out for. I urge mindfulness. See the previous page for instructions on how to do these and just do them sitting on the edge of the bed.

You can modify the Bear Hug by keeping your elbows bent when you throw your arms wide.

There is also a rather less energetic replacement for the Carnival Ride. Sit at the edge of your bed, legs hanging over, and lift your arms up parallel to the floor, straight in front of you. As you exhale swing your arms slowly to the right and twist your body as far around as possible in that direction. This allows you to adjust for any obstacles.

Inhale as you bring your arms back to the center, then exhale to the left as you did to the right. You can do this as many times as you like so long as you twist an equal number of times in each direction.

in the Bedroom

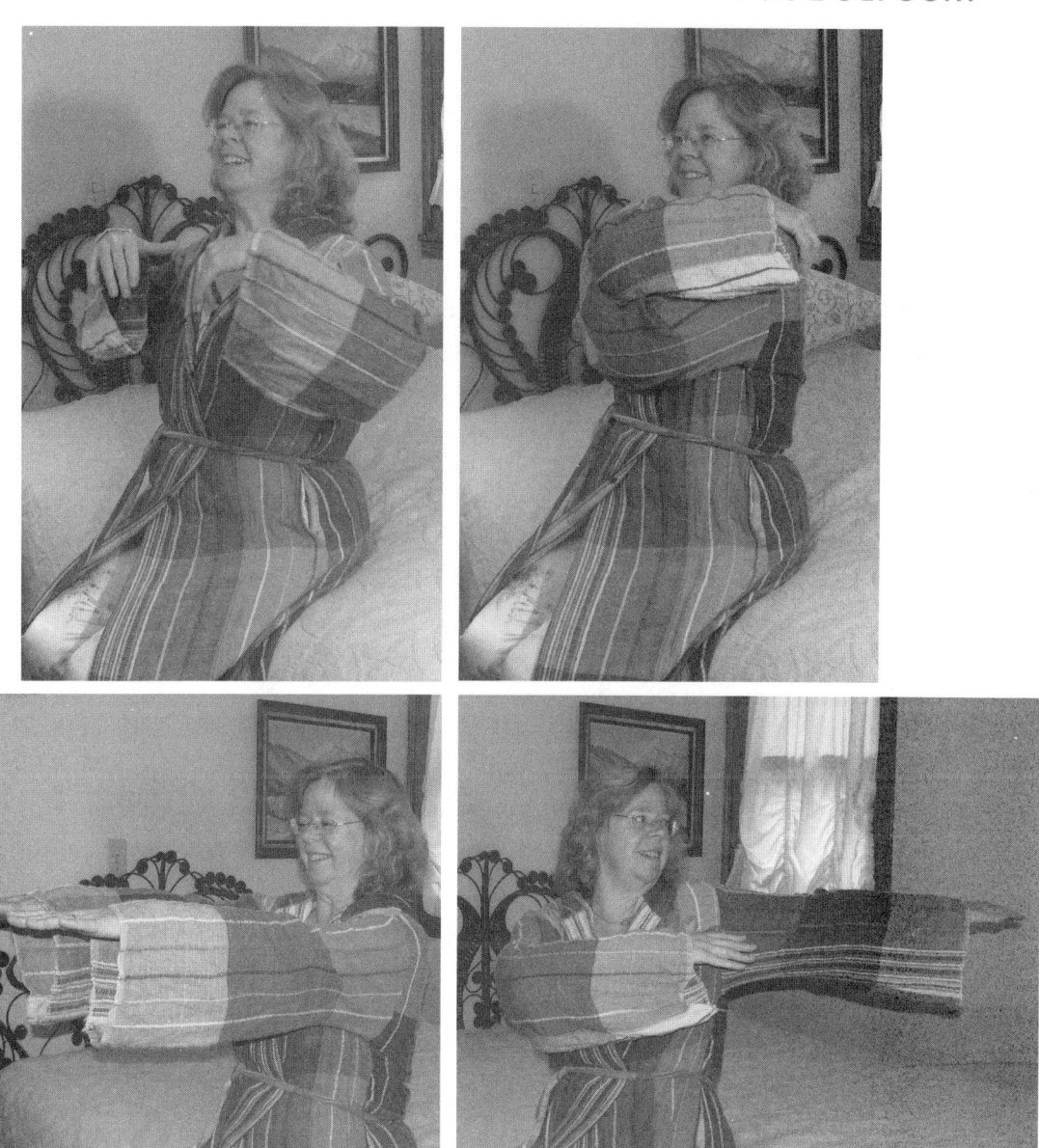

19

in the Bedroom

Neck Stretches

This is very helpful when there is pain in the neck and shoulders. It is helpful too, for beginning to build strength in the neck. Very valuable if you ever want to do headstands. Just don't do headstands before bed. They'll stimulate the brain cells rather than calm them. *It is particularly important to do this exercise mindfully and gently. Back off if anything hurts. Otherwise you're working against your goal.*

As you exhale, let your chin drop to your chest. If you're not feeling much stretch, press it into your chest slightly. Take two or three breaths in this position.

The next time you inhale, lift your head up and as you continue to inhale, drop your head back so that your chin is pointed at the ceiling (or as close as you can come to it—be gentle with yourself). Take another two or three breaths; then, as you exhale, lift your head back to its normal position.

Inhale and let your head fall gently toward a shoulder (without lifting either shoulder—try doing this in the bathroom in front of a mirror now and then so you can see whether you are unconsciously lifting a shoulder). Take two or three breaths in this position. The next time you inhale, lift your head to vertical. As you exhale again, let it fall gently toward your other shoulder (again, without lifting a shoulder). Take two or three more breaths before lifting your head back to vertical on an inhalation.

Keeping your head vertical and level, turn it gently to one side as far as it will go. Hold for two or three breaths. Turn it gently to the other side and hold for two or three breaths.

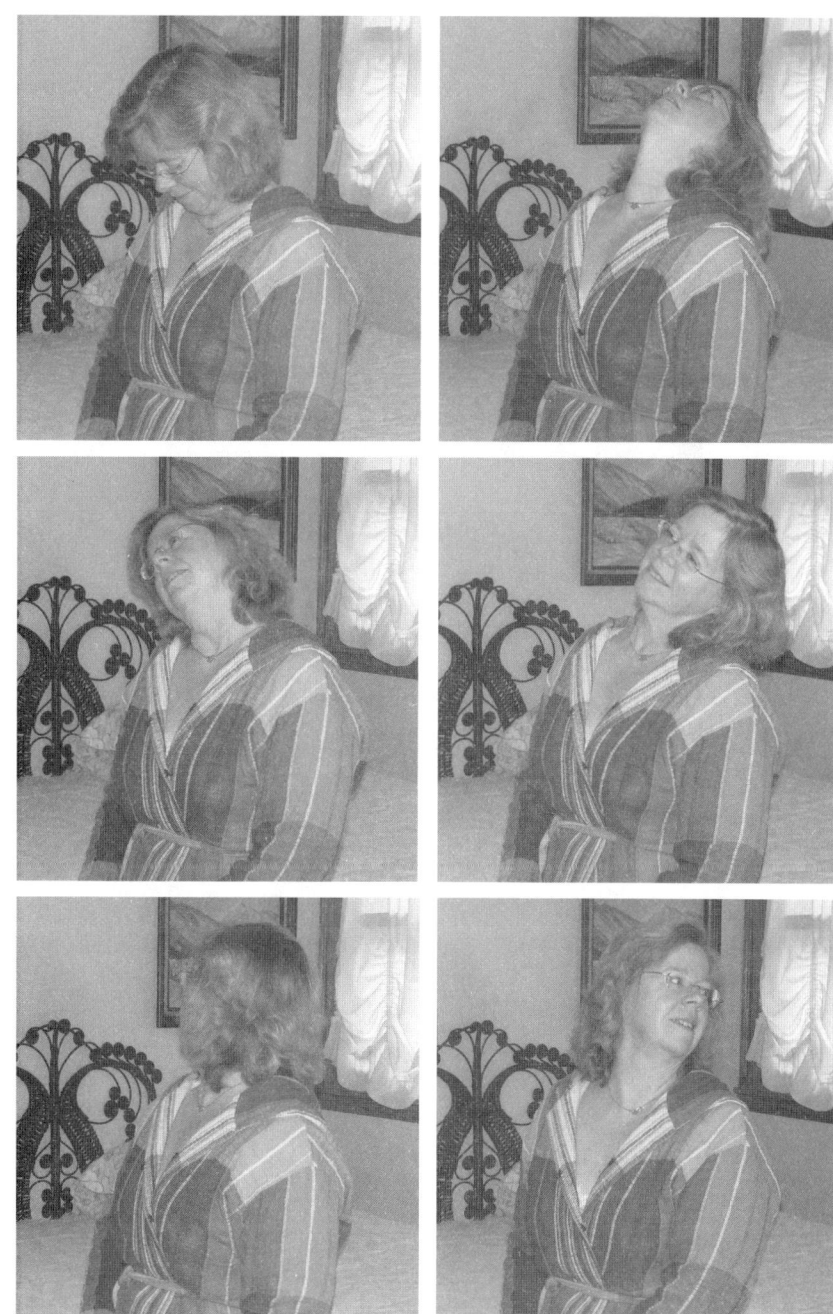

in the Bedroom

Shoulder Circles

Another beauty for loosening the shoulders and neck! Powerful stress reliever on those days when everything has been on your shoulders.

Begin by taking a deep breath, then, as you exhale, bring your shoulders forward. As you inhale, lift your shoulders up and back. Exhaling, circle your shoulders down and forward. Repeat three or four times in that direction, stopping with your shoulders in the forward position. Reverse direction. Inhale as the shoulders go down and back. Exhale as they go up and forward. Repeat three or four times.

Relax.

in the **Bedroom**

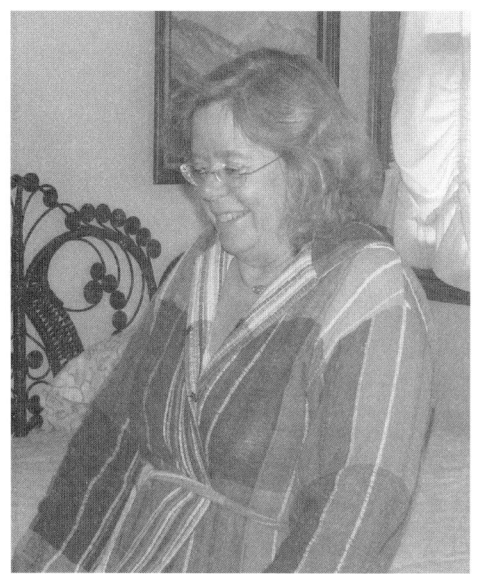

Up

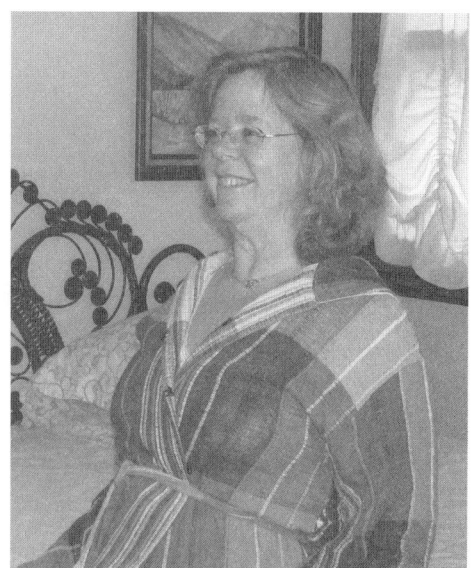

Back

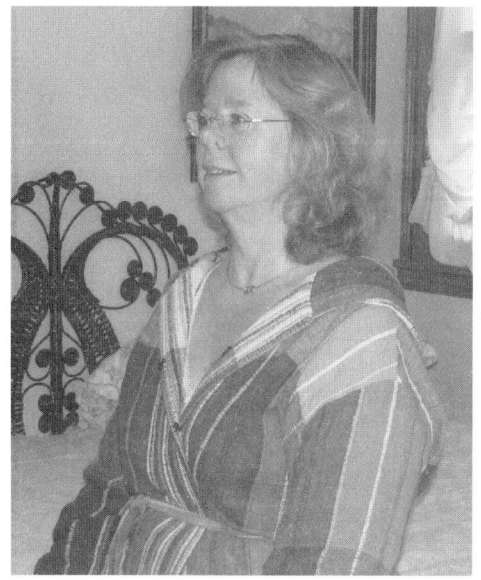

Down

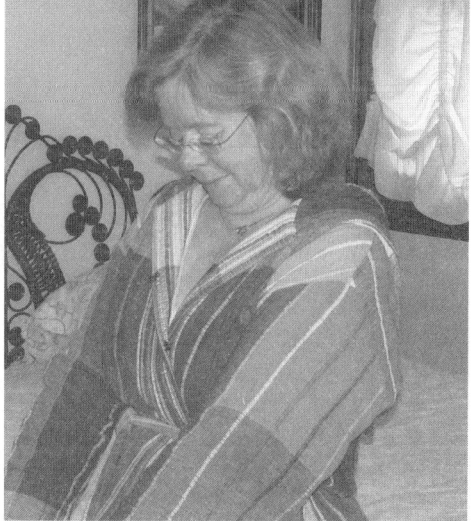

Forward

in the Bedroom

Chicken Arms

In case the shoulder circles didn't do enough for the huge amounts of tension you carry in the shoulder area, here's another exercise that helps. It is also really great for lubricating the shoulder joints.

As you inhale, lift your arms straight out to the sides. Turn your palms so they face up and bend your elbows so your fingertips touch your shoulders. Now, draw ten great big circles with your elbows. Then do ten in the other direction. Pay attention to all of the muscles and bones that cooperate in this movement.

Remember to back off at any sign of pain. A recent rotator cuff injury is an excellent reason to give this exercise the go-by.

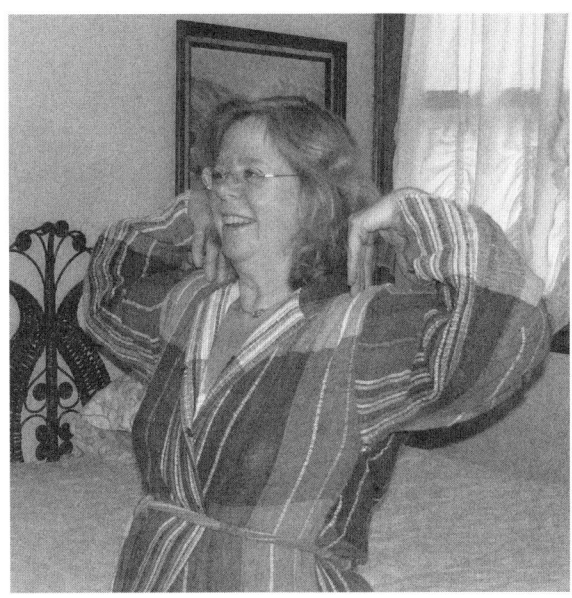

in the Bedroom

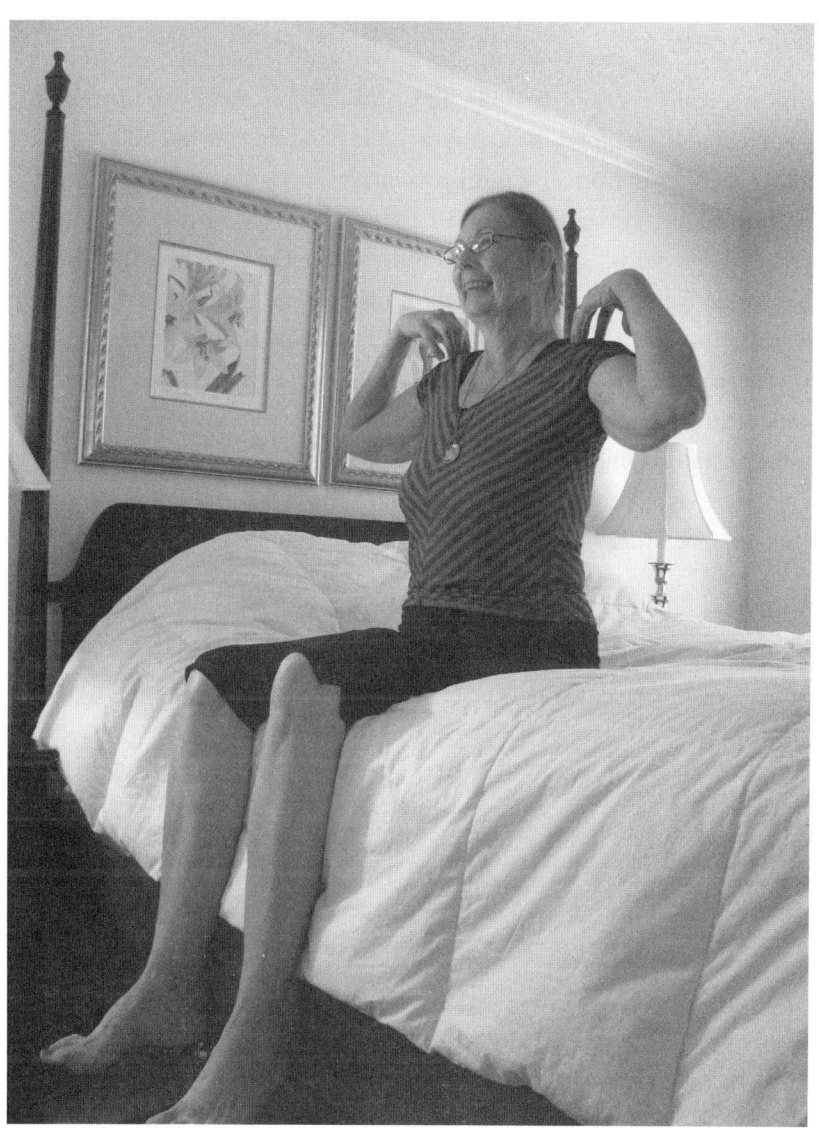

in the Bedroom

Side Bend

This is a really nice one to do in bed. Sitting comfortably on the edge of your bed and keeping hips level, rest your hand on the bed beside you and slide it away from you until you can rest your elbow on the bed. Arch the other arm over your head and reach with it toward the wall your head is pointing toward. You want to feel the stretch in the ribcage, not in the waist. Because we so seldom stretch the muscles between the ribs in our daily life, tight muscles here limit how deeply we can inhale. If we can't breathe deeply, we short-change ourselves in terms of general health. Stretching these muscles also releases tensions we may be unaware of carrying.

Take two or three deep breaths, then sit back up and do the same thing on the other side.

in the Bedroom

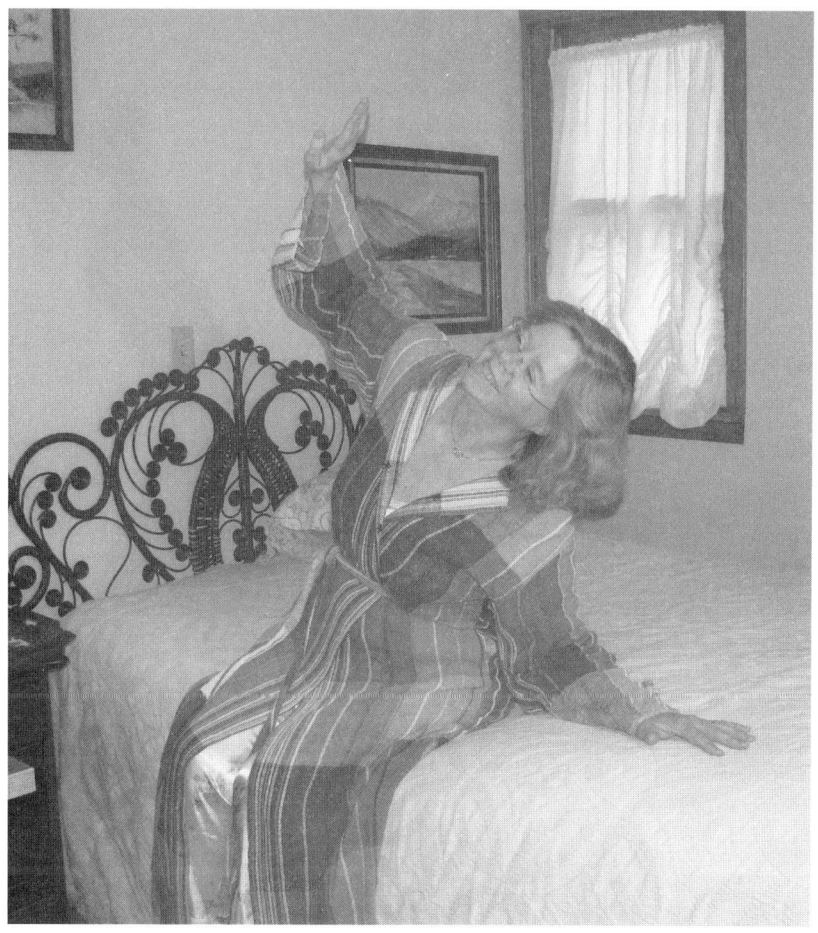

in the Bedroom

Forward Bend

Forward bends have a deeper meaning than the purely physical. The ease with which we do forward bends is an indicator of how well we are able to surrender in life. Control freaks have a tendency to have trouble with forward bends and when we're getting ready to sleep, being able to surrender that control is a potent ability. For this exercise, be sure you feel stable and supported. If your bed is too tall for that, try the couch.

Being supported by the bed is helpful in allowing just that little extra feeling of safety that makes bending forward less scary. So, sitting on the edge of your bed, plant your feet solidly on the floor (if your bed is too tall for your feet to touch the floor, sit back as far as you can and still have your legs hang over the edge) and spread your feet and knees far enough apart that your chest can fit between your knees. Inhaling, lift your arms up over your head. Exhaling, keep your arms extended and bend forward from the hips while keeping your back straight as far as possible. Then, let everything relax and hang down between your knees.

Take several deep breaths and every time you exhale, be conscious of relaxing a fraction of an inch farther forward.

Place your hands on top of your knees. Push yourself back up to a sitting position on an inhalation.

in the Bedroom

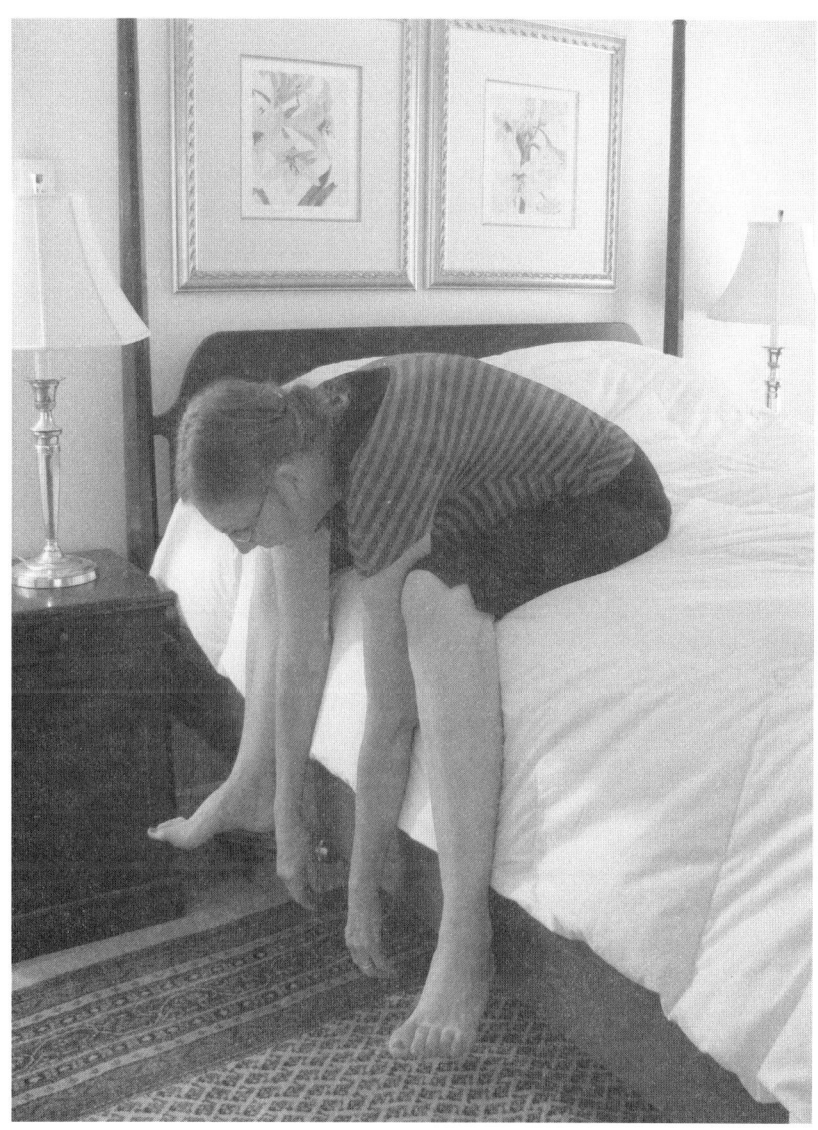

29

in the Bedroom

Backbend

After a forward bend, we need to balance the body by bending backwards. And backbends offer their own challenges. Those of us who have trouble with bending backwards also tend to have difficulty trusting the world, other people, God, the Great Spirit and All That Is. Sometimes sleep is elusive because we don't quite trust either sleep or dreaming, or because we don't quite trust the world we call reality to not let us down while we're sleeping. Cultivating a healthy backbend can help.

Doing the backbend while seated on the edge of a bed can boost your confidence because you simply cannot fall down.

Start out by placing your hands on the mattress just slightly behind your hips. As you inhale, lift your chest toward the ceiling and lean backward on your hands. Gently bend your elbows until you are supported by them. Let your head drop back and breathe several deep breaths.

Sit back up, pushing off with your hands on an exhalation.

in the **Bedroom**

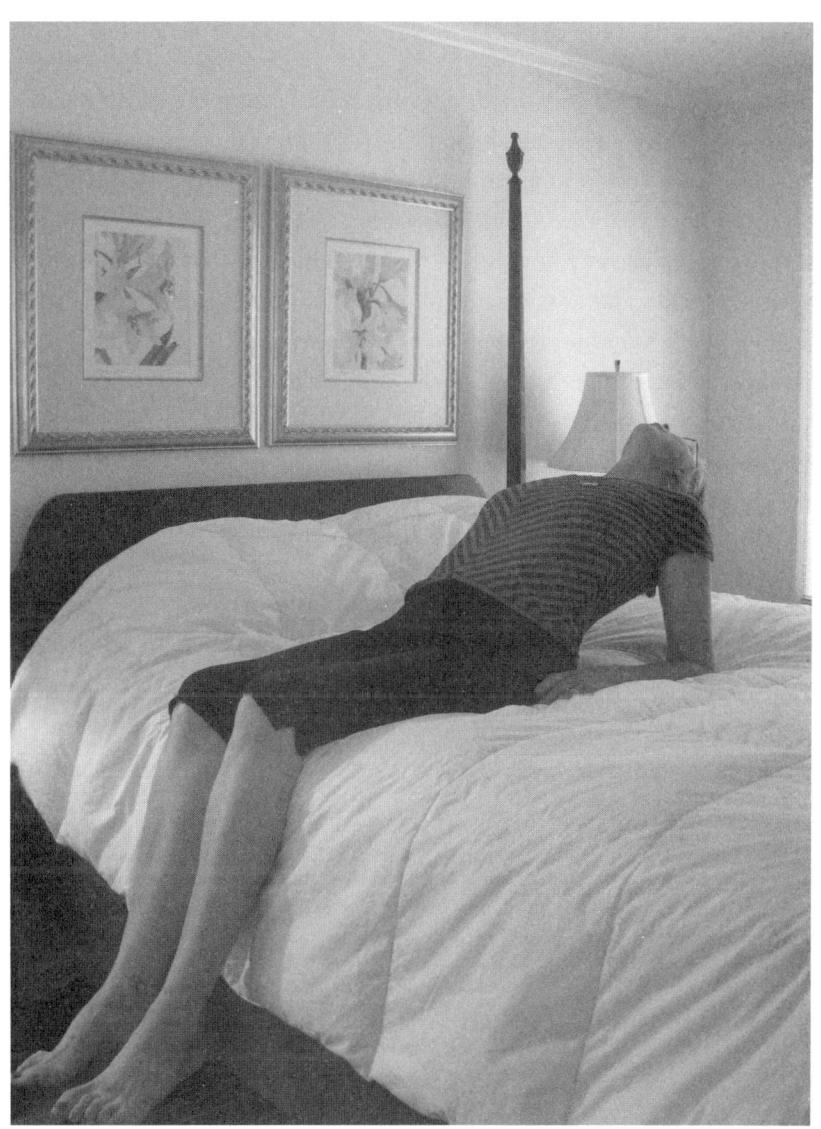

in the Bedroom

Twisting, Turning . . .

This is another nice exercise for releasing tension from the back. In addition, it provides a three-step benefit for your internal organs.

From your comfortable position seated on the edge of your bed, place your right hand on the outside of your left knee. Inhale to lengthen your spine, then exhale as you twist your body to the left. Reach behind with your left hand as far as you can and place it on the mattress (your hips stay planted). Use it for leverage to help you twist even more deeply in that direction. Turn your head in the same direction. Hold this position for two or three breaths and, inhaling, relax back to the front. Make sure you take those deep, full breaths we talked about earlier. They make all the difference. Do the same thing in the opposite direction.

in the Bedroom

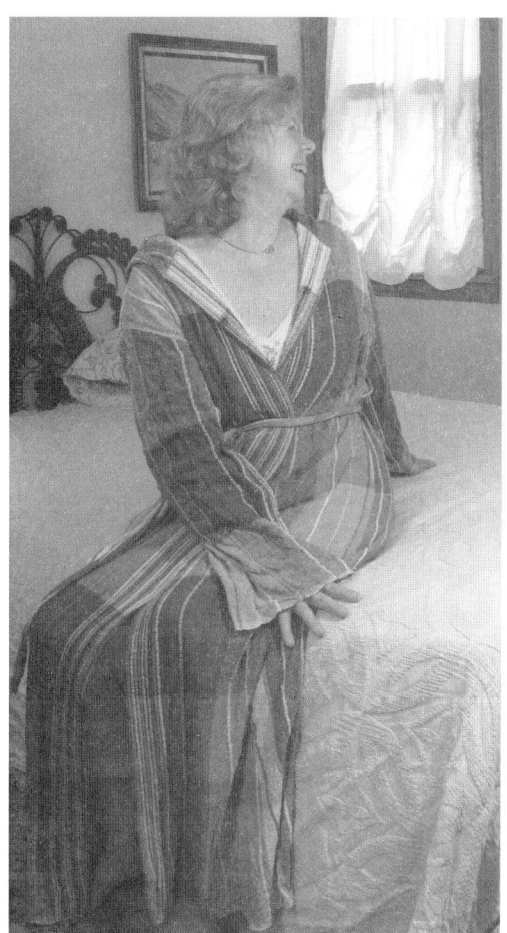
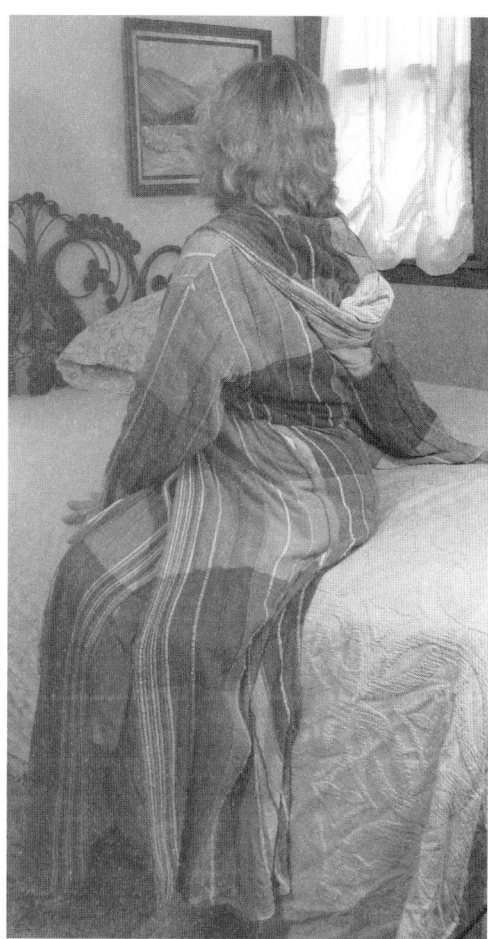

in the Bedroom

Flat on Your Back

Once you've done all the seated poses you can handle, it's time to lie down. Lie on your back and just relax for a moment or two.

If you drift off to sleep, great! If you are still wakeful, here are a few more exercises to work with. You can do them in any order that seems attractive, and give yourself an opportunity to fall asleep after each. Set your pillow aside while you do them.

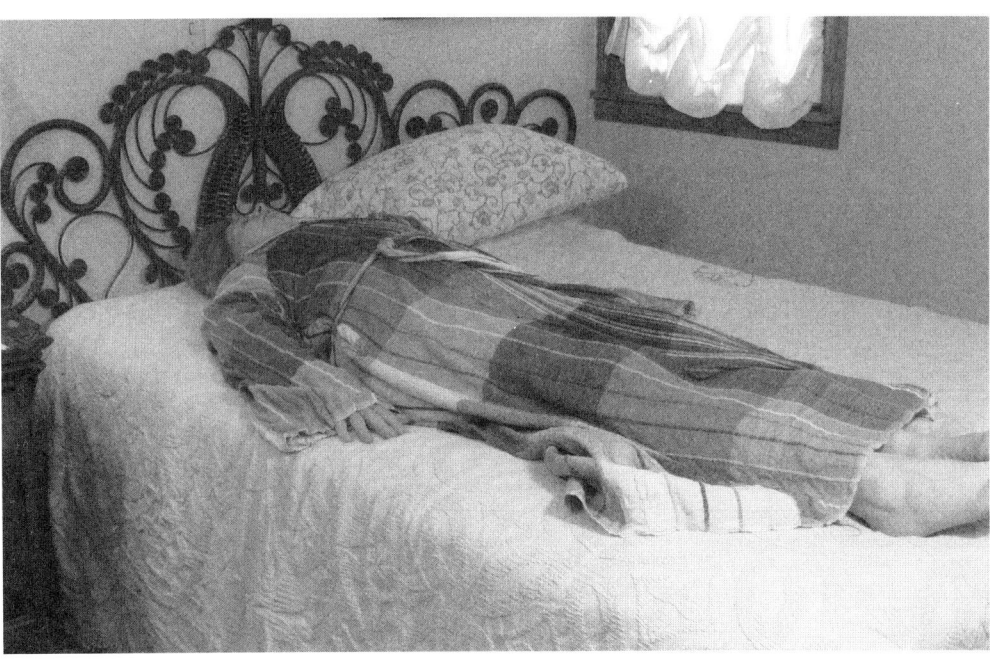

in the **Bedroom**

Hamstring Stretch

I used to hate this one when my yoga teacher made us do it at the end of every class just before the meditation. What I discovered as time went on is that if I did it in bed before sleep it was very good for short-circuiting the kind of insomnia characterized by bodily restlessness. Students of mine who get the spasm type of charley horse when trying to fall asleep have found that a good hamstring stretch reduces them almost to zero.

In addition to the sleep-encouraging benefits of hamstring stretches, there are other important benefits. Chief among them is that tight hamstrings flatten the curve of the lower back. This diminishes its stability and leaves it vulnerable to injury. Hamstrings do need to be strong, for good back health, but not tight.

1. As you lie on your back, pay attention to how your body feels from top to bottom. Next bend your knees so your feet are side-by-side up close to your body. Lift one foot up off the bed and straighten the leg so the toe points at the ceiling. Bend it and straighten it three times.

2. With your leg straight up and your foot high in the air, do three or four ankle circles both clockwise and counter-clockwise. Flex your foot up tight (creating an acute angle between ankle and foot), then point your toe. Repeat this back and forth three or four times. Relax your ankle.

3. Now, leg still straight and foot still high in the air, if you can reach your ankle with your hands (keeping your leg straight) do so. Otherwise get a scarf, a neck-tie or a belt and loop it behind your ankle (not across the bottom of your foot). I like to keep a nice Guatemalan woven belt for this purpose. Silk feels good too. Push away with the leg (imagine pressing the back of your knee toward the opposite wall) while you pull

in the Bedroom

with your arms. Your leg is being encouraged to straighten. Take three or four deep breaths. Release the ankle but keep the leg in the air.

4. Cock your foot up tight and keeping it cocked, slowly lower your leg (keeping it straight) almost to the mattress. Stop with your foot about three inches up off the mattress and do three or four ankle circles in both directions. Flex your foot up tight (creating an acute angle between ankle and foot), then point your toe back and forth three or four times. Then, keeping it cocked up tight again, lift your leg all the way back up as you exhale. Repeat Step 3 again. This repeat wrings the last bit of tension out of your leg.

5. With cocked foot and straight leg, lower your leg slowly all the way down to the mattress. Bend your knee so your feet are side-by-side again and relax. Compare how your body feels now to how it felt the last time you checked in. Compare the right and left sides of your body and note any differences.

6. Repeat Steps 1 through 5 with the other leg.

Relax and give yourself a chance to fall asleep.

in the Bedroom

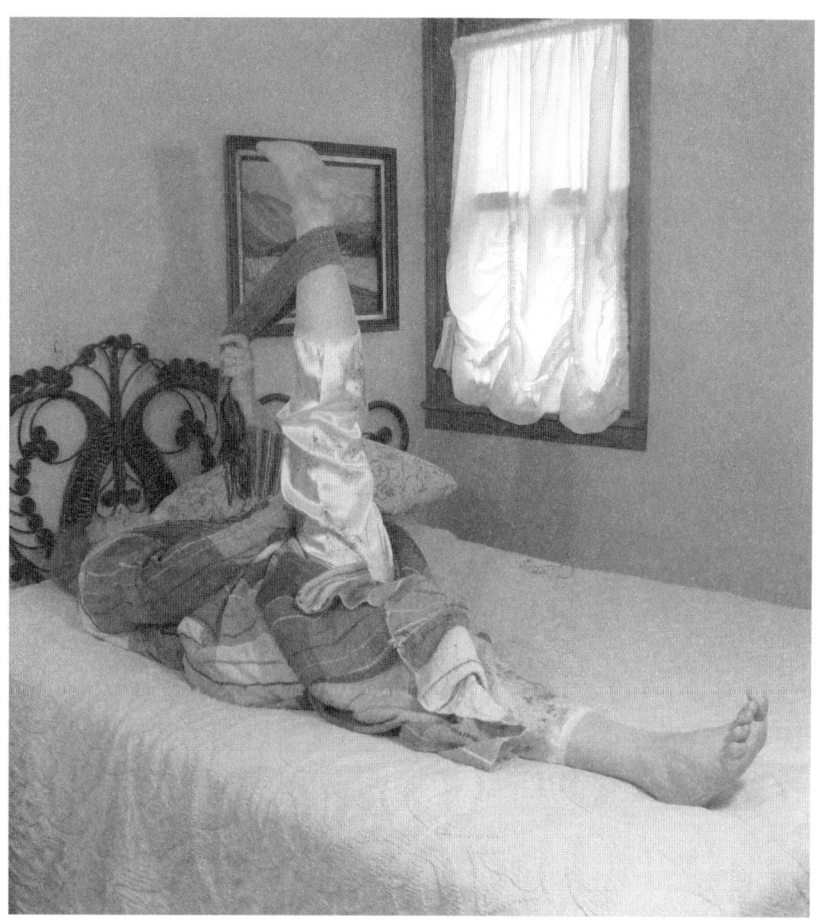

in the Bedroom

Toe-Grabbing Fun

If the hamstring stretch sounds like more than you can handle on any given night, this less complex alternative might help. The stretch isn't as intense, but intensity may not always be what you need.

Lie on your back with your knees bent and your feet up close to your body. Lift your feet up off the bed keeping your knees bent and reach through between your thighs to grab hold of your big toes with your first two fingers.

At first, keep your knees bent as you pull on your toes. This can give the lower back a gentle stretch. Next, keep a firm grasp on your big toes as you gently straighten your legs, pulling them together while pushing the backs of your knees toward the opposite wall. Take a few deep breaths as you hold this position.

Maintain your hold on your toes, keep your legs straight and let your legs separate and fall out to the side. Take a few deep breaths as you hold this position.

Bend your knees, release your toes and relax as you bring your feet back to the mattress.

This provides a gentle stretch to your hamstrings and Achilles tendon.

in the **Bedroom**

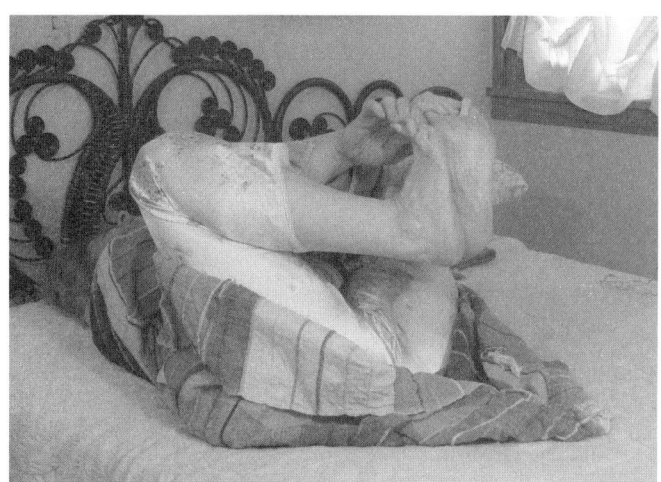
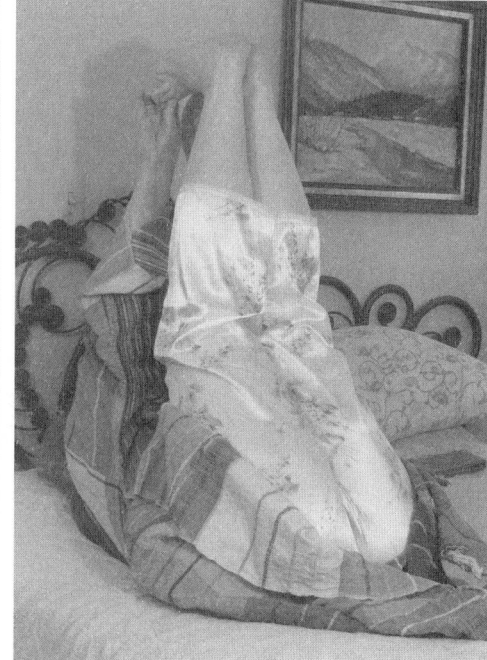
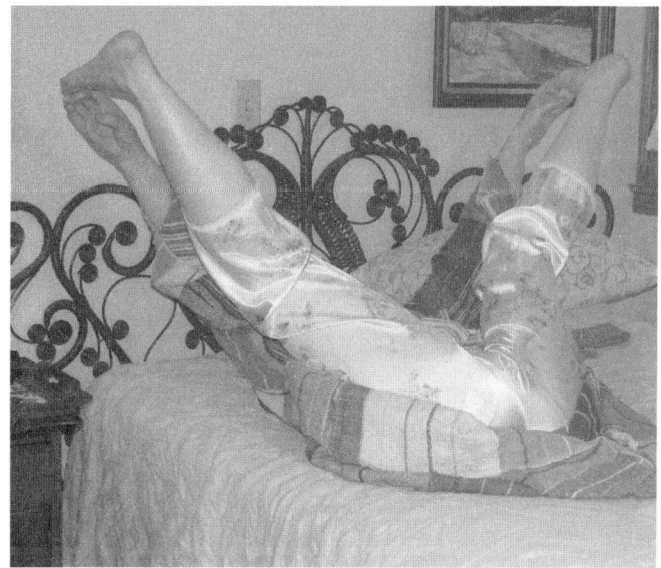

39

in the Bedroom

Cross Your Legs

Sometimes the outside of the hips can be so tight it's painful. This is a lovely, low-stress way to release some of that tension.

Lie on your back with both knees bent and your feet up close to your body. Place your right foot on the left thigh. Lift the left foot up off the bed. Use both hands to grab the left thigh just under the knee or reach over your right leg to grab the bent left knee from above—whichever is most comfortable for you. You can even loop a belt or scarf either around or under the left thigh if grabbing with your hands is uncomfortable. Take two or three deep breaths and imagine the breath is going straight to the place where you're feeling the tension.

Switch leg positions and repeat.

in the **Bedroom**

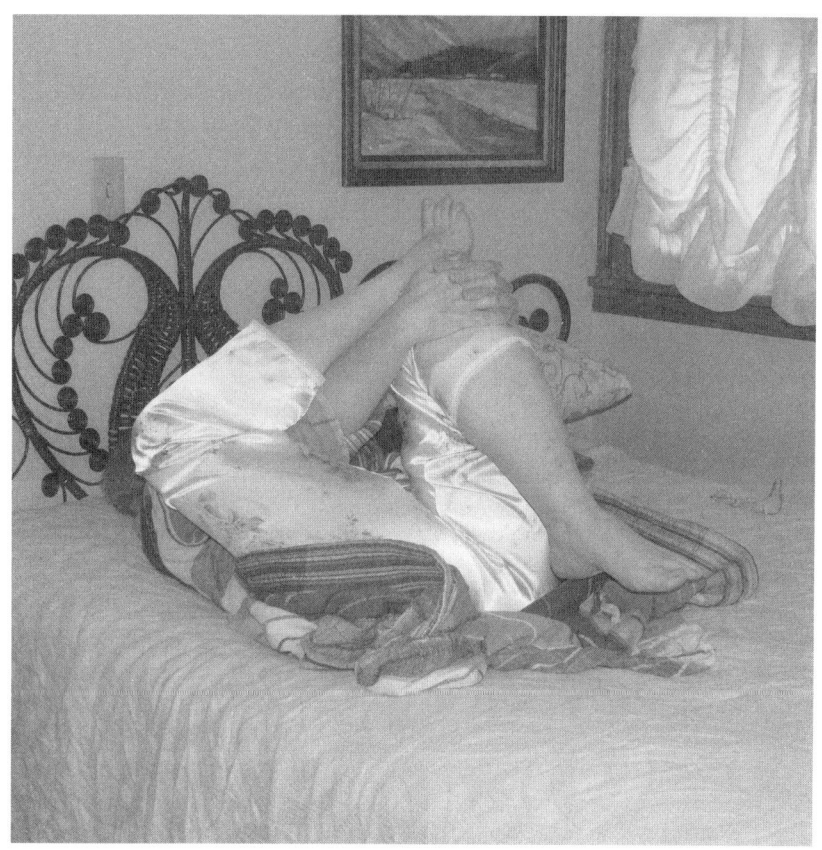

41

in the Bedroom

Restorative Pose

At the end of a long day of struggling to deal with the chaotic world of humanity, this pose can help you let go of it all and gently make the transition to sleep. It takes a bit of setup, but the rewards are lovely.

Well, maybe not so much setup if you already own a bolster. If you don't own such a thing, you can fold blankets to form a bolster a little narrower than your shoulders and long enough to reach from your waist to the top of your head. It should be three to five inches deep, depending on your body's proportions.

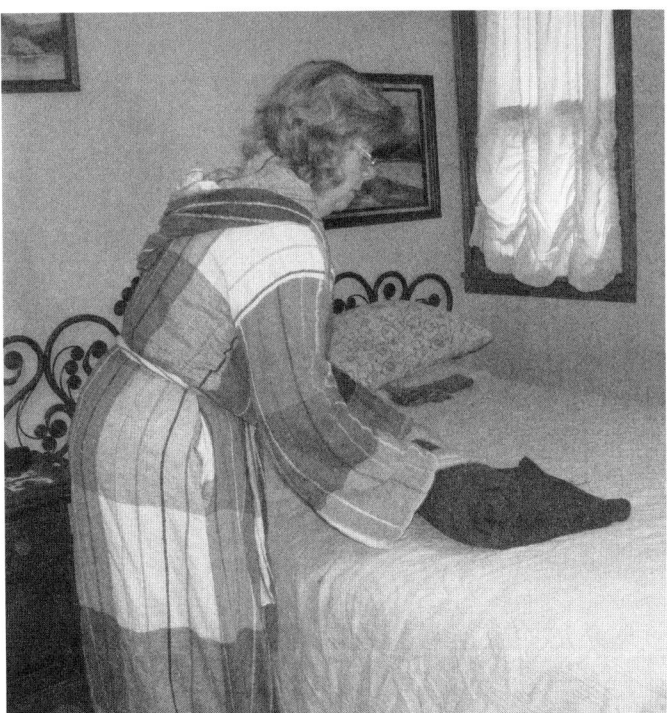

Position it lengthwise beneath your ribcage with one end touching your lower back so that it can also support your head. Relax, let your shoulders fall back around the bolster with your arms resting palms up beside your body. Breathe deeply and slowly.

This pose opens the chest and relieves tension.

Rolling blanket into bolster shape

in the **Bedroom**

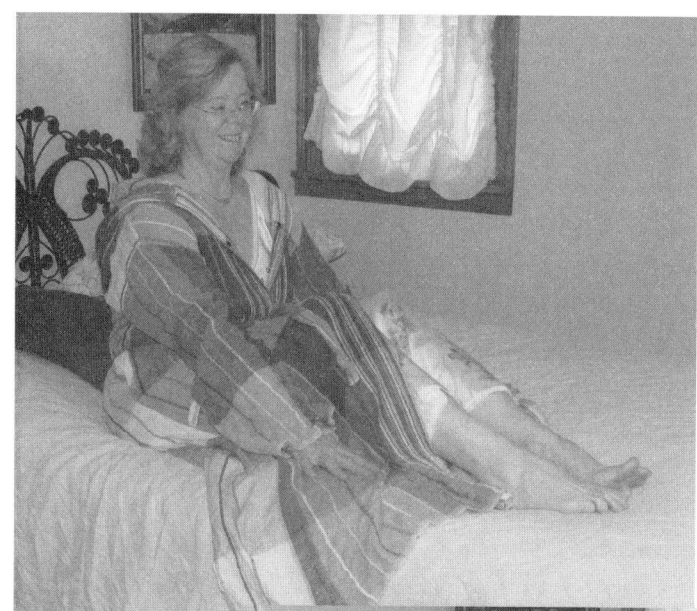

Bolster placement

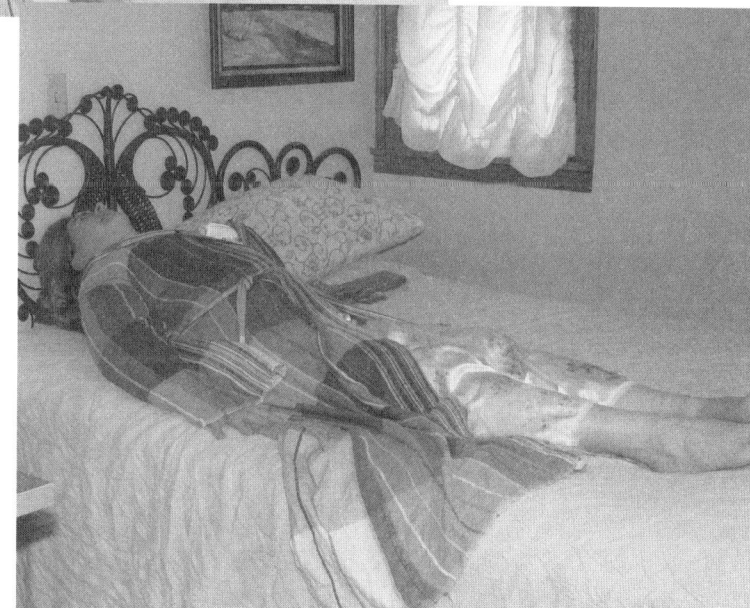

Lying on bolster

in the Bedroom

Legs Up the Wall

This is another restorative pose for the end of a stressful day, particularly if you've been on your feet a long time. You can also do this on the floor.

Sit sidewise on the bed so one hip is touching the nearest wall (or the head of the bed). Swivel around so your back is flat on the bed and your legs are extended upward flat against the wall. Both cheeks of your shapely behind should be touching (or as close to it as you can possibly get them) the wall or the headboard.

If your bed is located far from any wall, you'll have to improvise. If you don't mind lying on the floor you can cosy up to any old wall to do this. Another alternative is to sit on the floor facing a chair. Your legs should be on either side of the chair. Scootch your hips up close to the chair legs and lie back, simply resting your calves in the seat. You can stay in this position 10 or 15 minutes with your legs either up the wall or on the chair seat.

in the Bedroom

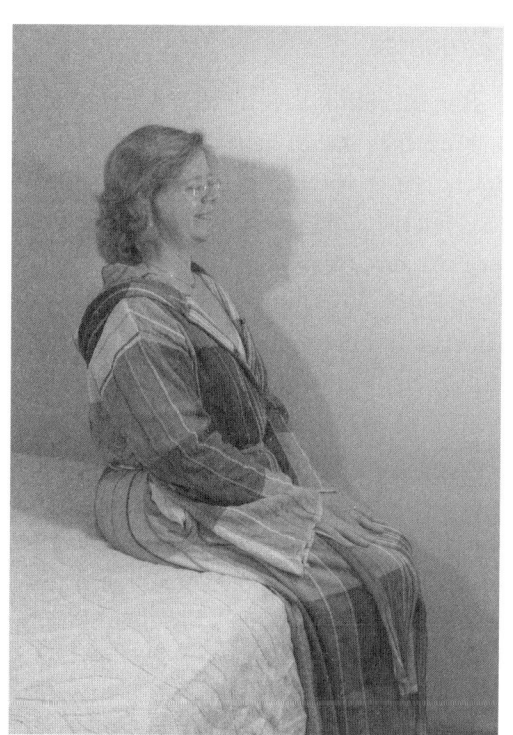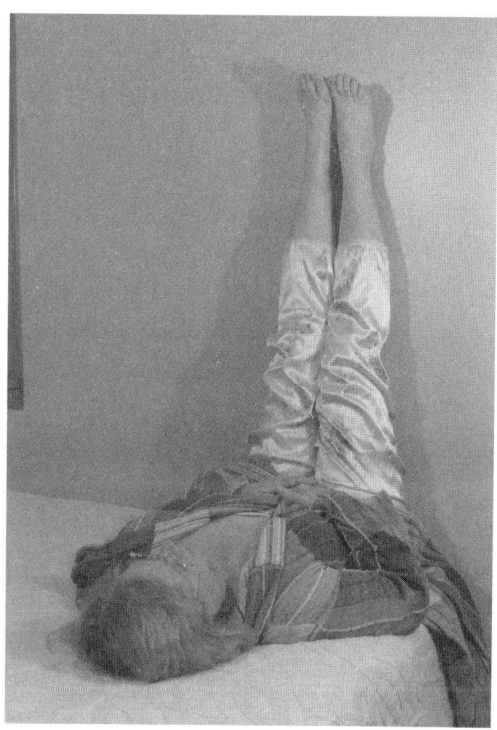

in the Bedroom

Face Massage—Sweet Dreams

Have you ever looked at yourself in the mirror after a tough day and seen those vertical lines on your forehead, the pinched look around your mouth and eyes? And when you lie down to sleep has your body felt willing but your head, particularly your face, felt tight and screwed up as though prepared for opposition? On those occasions, try this facial massage.

Place the fleshy pads at the base of your thumbs on either side of the bridge of your nose. Fingers and thumbs point up to begin. Palms are facing one another. Pressing firmly, but gently, trace the curve of your face up alongside your nose and all the way around the top and outside edges of your eye sockets with the pad at the base of your thumb. At the end of the arc your fingers should be pointing downward and the pad at the base of your thumb pressing gently against the front edge of your temple. Bringing your hands back to the starting position and using the same kind of motion, complete a slightly larger circle, this time running those fleshy pads up and around, just above the eye sockets. Continue this pattern making each circuit run a little higher on your forehead until you reach your hairline.

To massage the lower half of your face, position your hands so that the fleshy parts at the bases of your thumbs are again against the nose, but now the thumbs and fingers are pointed downward and outward. Apply gentle pressure through the base of your thumbs without touching your eyes or eyelids. Maintain this pressure as you swivel your hands around your eyes along the eye socket. Continue this motion, massaging successive circuits of your lower face a little farther down each time. The final circuit follows the edge of your jaw.

in the **Bedroom**

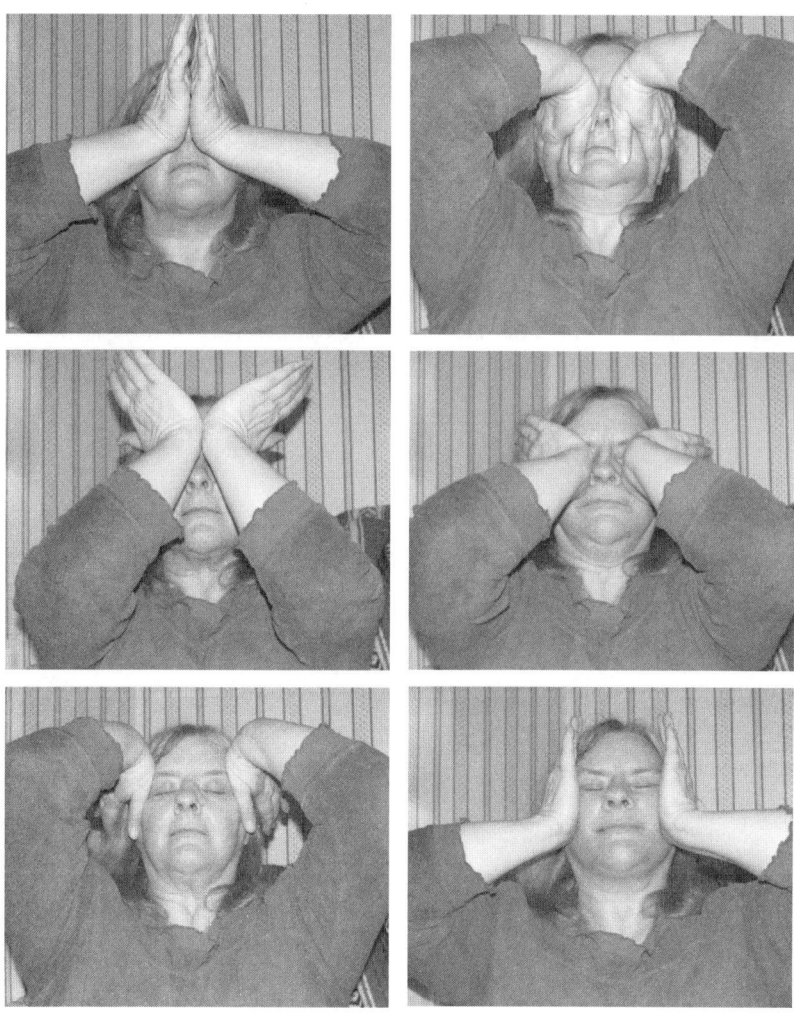

Upper face *Lower face*

in the **Bedroom**

If All Else Fails, Meditate

The simplest way to meditate is to follow the movement of breath in your body. Pay close attention to what it feels like to inhale. Notice the point at which your breath turns and you begin to exhale. Follow the breath all the way out to the point where it turns and you begin to inhale again. As you continue to breathe and pay attention to your breath, let that breath carry you deeper and deeper inside yourself. Let go of your consciousness of your body, the temperature of the room, and any sounds that might distract you. Just breathe. Let your body relax. Go to sleep.

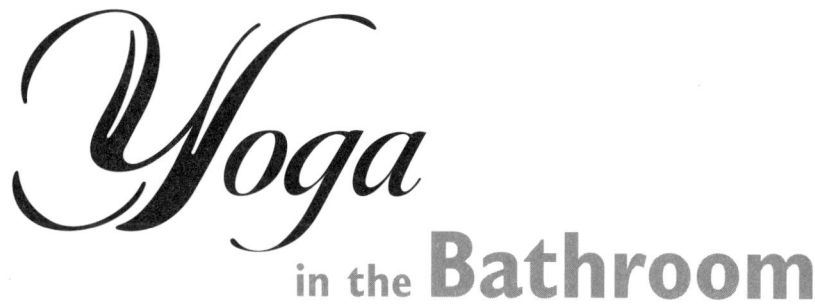

Yoga in the Bathroom

There are a number of poses that can be transferred to the bathroom. For instance, the seated twisted pose can be adapted for the toilet, as can the seated forward and back bends. Be creative. Each bathroom lends itself to different poses. See what works in yours.

in the Bathroom

Cow Face Pose

I suppose it had to be called something. It stretches parts of the upper arms that don't normally get much stretching. It also helps open the chest, and counteracts the tendency of shoulders to round as we age.

While standing in the tub if you're taking a shower, or sitting in the tub if taking a bath, start by stretching one arm toward the sky, then bend your elbow so the forearm and hand dangle down behind your head. With the other hand reach behind your back and up with your palm out until the hands meet and can clasp one another. If they don't touch, dangle a wash cloth or towel from the upper hand to bridge the distance and work your hands as close together as possible.

Hold the position for a few breaths and then switch arms. Doing this one regularly reduces your need for a loofah on a stick. Eventually you'll be able to reach your whole back without it!

in the Bathroom

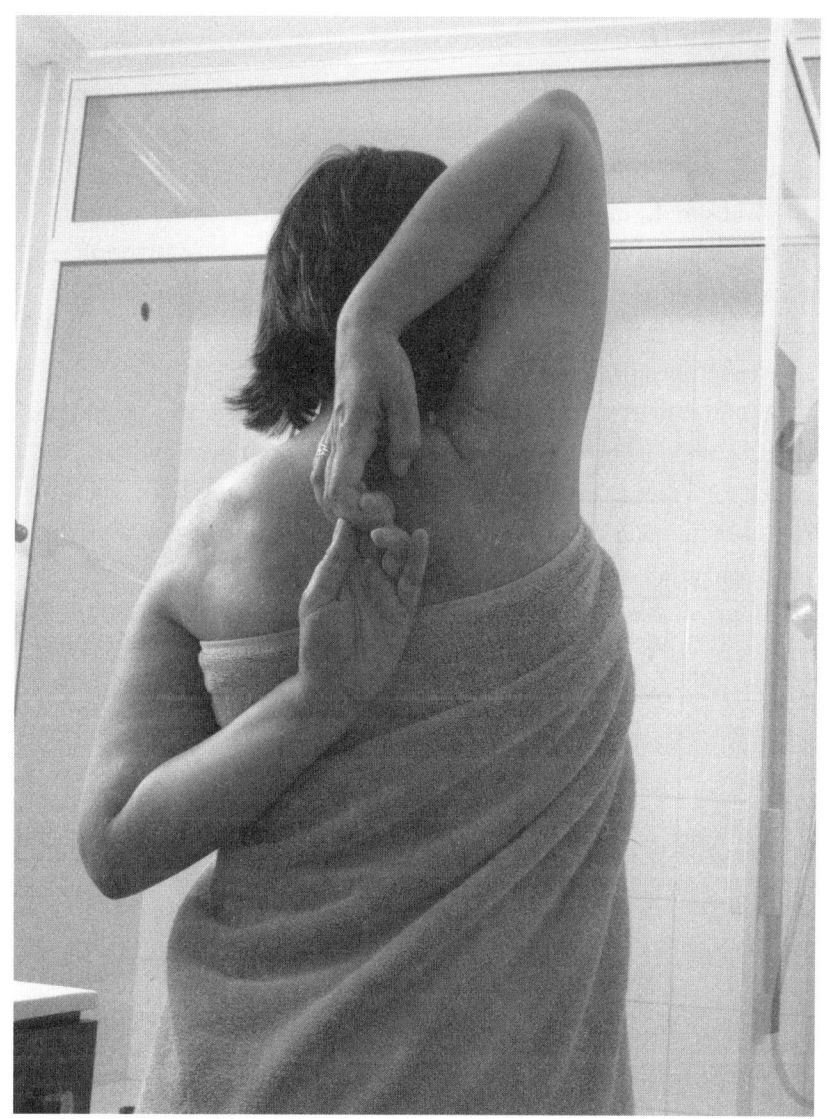

in the Bathroom

Cat on the Tub

While you're waiting for the hot water to make its way from the hot water heater to the tub, stand with your feet at least an arm's length away from the tub. Bend over and rest your hands on the side of the tub. You should now be in a roughly table-shaped position (allowing for the amazing variety of body shapes and sizes—not to mention relative tub heights). If your hands are not directly below your shoulders and your feet are not directly below your hips, adjust the position of your feet appropriately.

As you exhale, picture the way an angry cat's back arches up and press the back of your spine toward the ceiling. Tuck your head and hold the stretch for a few seconds. Then, as you inhale, relax your back and allow your belly to hang down—like a sway-backed old horse—while lifting your head and looking upward.

Alternate these positions in synch with your breath while the tub fills.

in the Bathroom

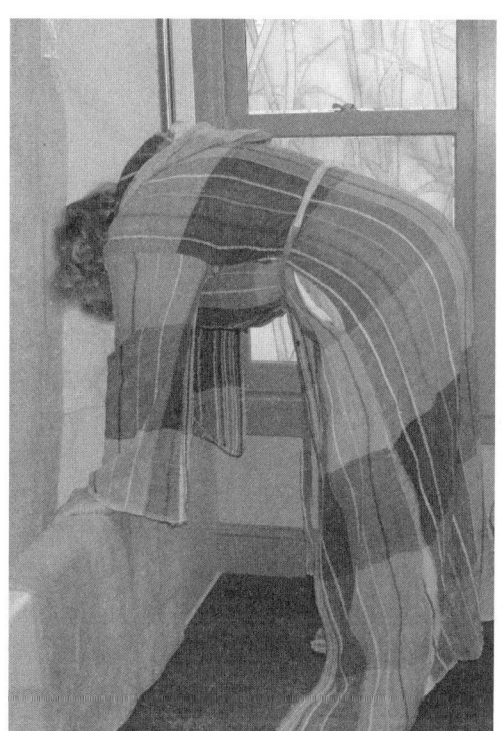
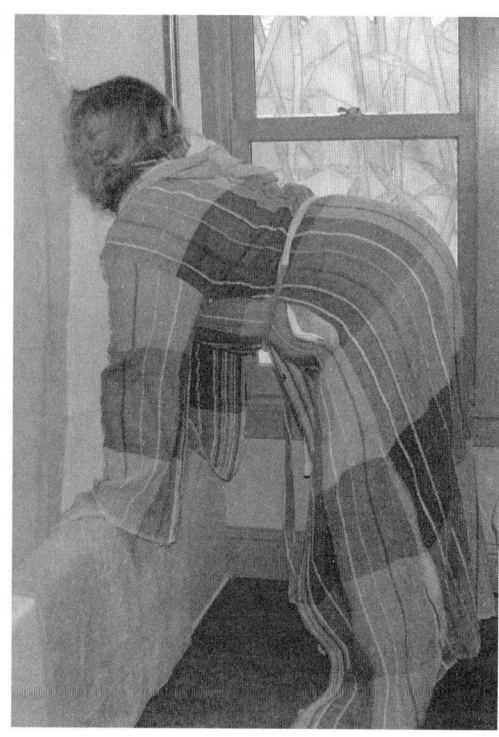

in the Bathroom

Bathing the Kids Squat

One of the worst inventions of humankind is the chair. Originally, only kings sat in chairs and enjoyed the attendant maladies of constipation, gas, and decreased flexibility. As time went on, other folks thought they were as good as kings (or, at least, better than peasants) and started sitting in chairs. In cultures where chairs are uncommon, so is milk of magnesia.

A good way to counteract the ills engendered by chairs is the humble squat. It starts out difficult for some people, but, little by little, squatting by the tub to wash squirming, bouncing, energetic young-uns, or simply to stretch vital areas, will bring more flexibility, better digestion, and softer stools. You'll feel like a kid yourself! If you have a condition affecting the knees, check with your most trusted expert before squatting.

Start out facing the tub, holding its edge for stability and to keep you from over-squatting. With your feet a bit more than shoulder width apart, bend at hips and knees gently until you feel a stretch. If it starts to feel scary, back off. At first, you may not be able to do this and keep your heels on the floor. That's okay. Do the best you can. Work at this a little every day. One day, you'll be able to squat comfortably without the aid of the tub.

Another approach is to bring your hands to the floor between your feet and use your elbows to brace your knees as you lower your hips. This one you can do anywhere! See which way works best for you.

in the Bathroom

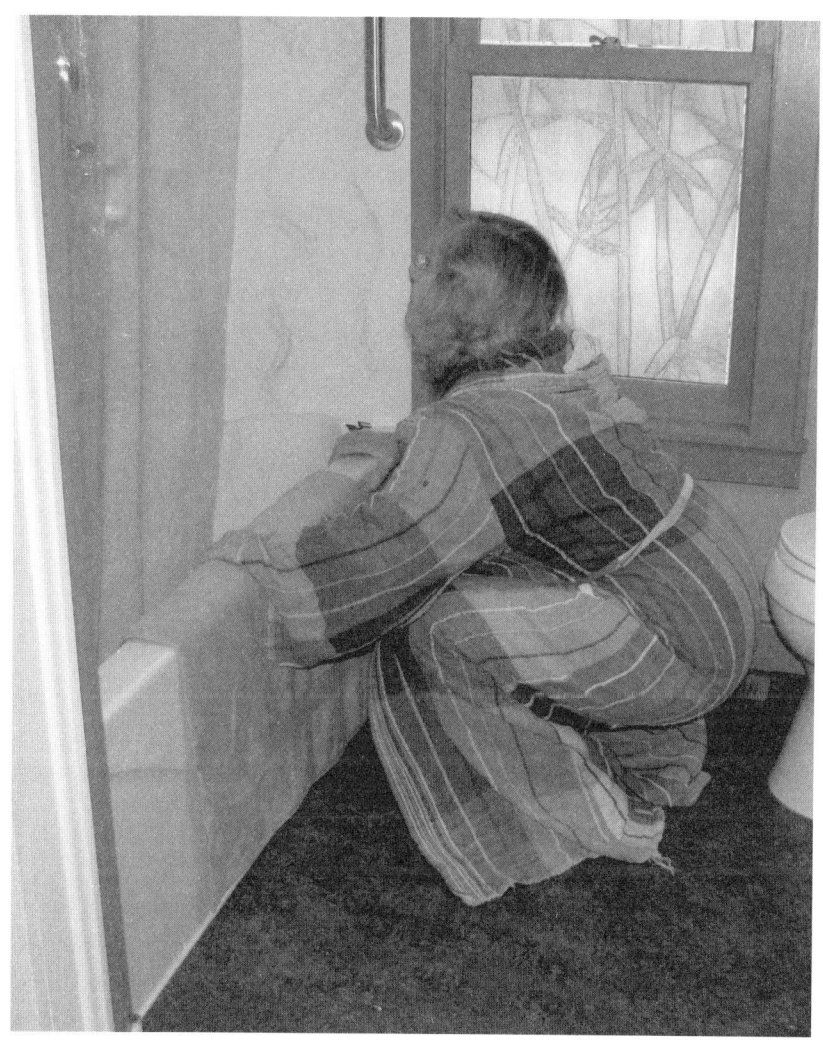

in the Bathroom

The Neti Pot

The neti pot is a small pitcher with a long thin spout used to rinse nasal passages. It helps fight airborne illnesses and minimizes nasal allergies. Some drugstores carry neti pots, but not all. You can use a large baby's medicine dropper instead. Fill the pot or syringe with warm, salty water (don't use sea salt if you're are allergic to shell-fish; you can use plain table salt) with a pinch of baking soda to soften the water. Lean forward over the basin and tilt your head to one side. Pour the water in one nostril. Let the water run out the other nostril. Rinse both nostrils three or four times. You can find numerous illustrative videos on YouTube®!

in the Bathroom

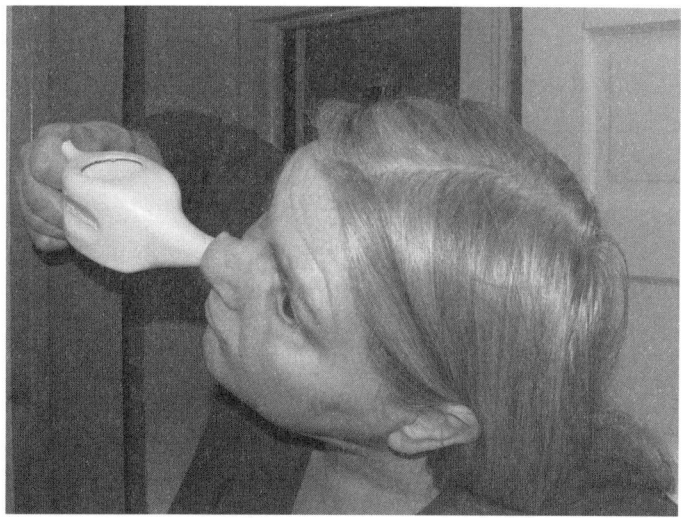

If the camera had waited just one more second you would have seen a stream of water issuing from the lower nostril!

in the Bathroom

Twisting, Turning . . . Reprise

From your comfortable position seated on the toilet, place your right hand on the outside of your left knee. Inhale as you lengthen your spine, then exhale as you twist your body to the left. Reach behind your body with your left hand as far as you can. Turn your head in the same direction as far as it will go. Hold this position for two or three deep, full breaths and inhale as you relax back to the front. Do the same thing turning toward the right.

in the Bathroom

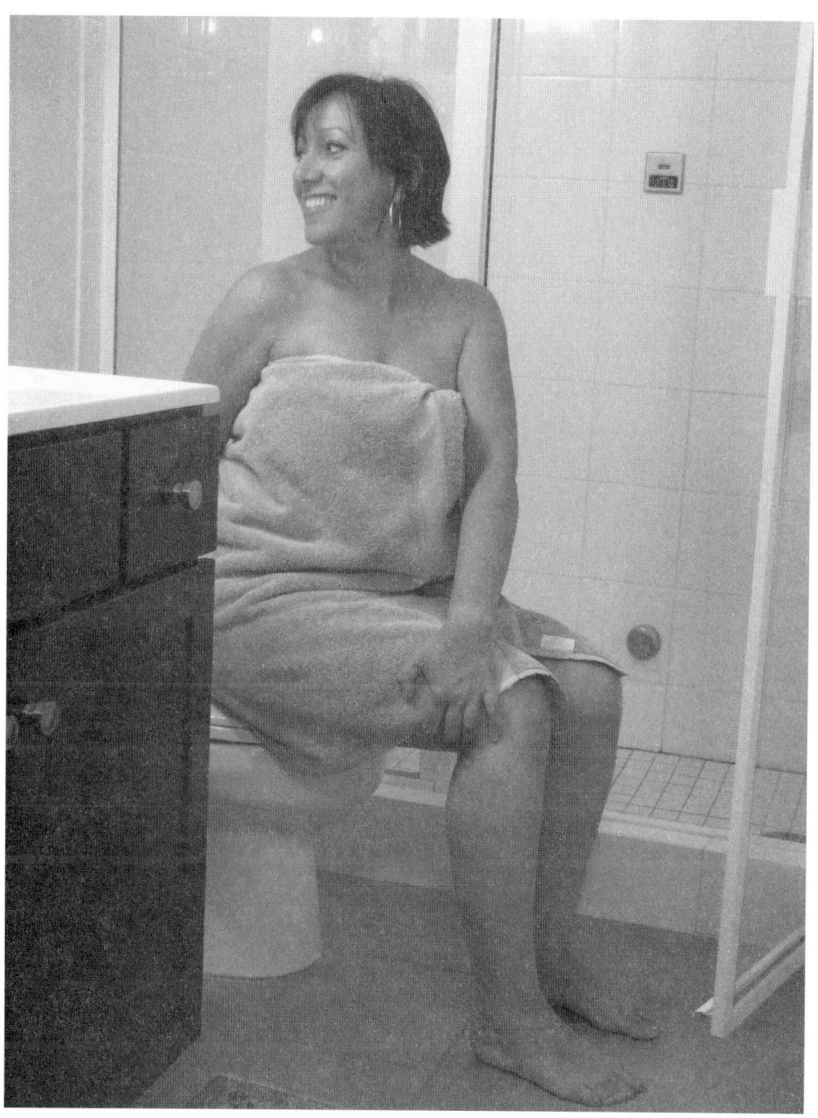

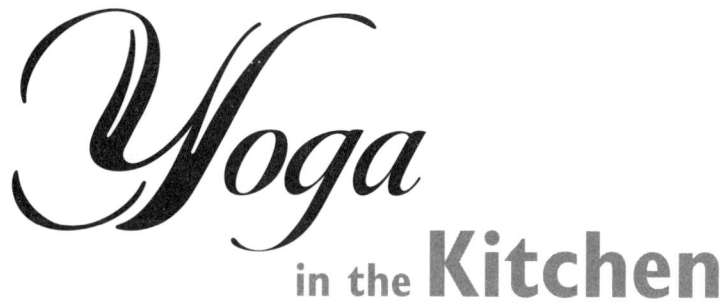

Yoga in the Kitchen

or "Things to Do While You Wait for the Water to Boil"

The kitchen is a great place to do yoga! There is so much waiting: waiting for water to boil, waiting for the roast to brown, waiting for the teenager or spouse to get his or her head out of the fridge so you can grab the roast and get it started browning . . .

The trick is to remember there is yoga you could be doing!

in the Kitchen

Mountain Pose and Meditation

Stand strong with your feet parallel to one another and shoulder width apart. Let your arms hang alongside your body. Find your center of balance (you can sway slightly to help locate it). Imagine roots growing out of your feet to anchor you in the earth itself. Breathe deeply and slowly, letting the breath carry you deep into your own center. Make no plans. Review nothing, neither past events nor future expectations. Be wholly present in the moment until the water boils.

The mountain pose helps you feel your own strength and your connection to the earth. It is the starting position for most of the standing poses.

in the Kitchen

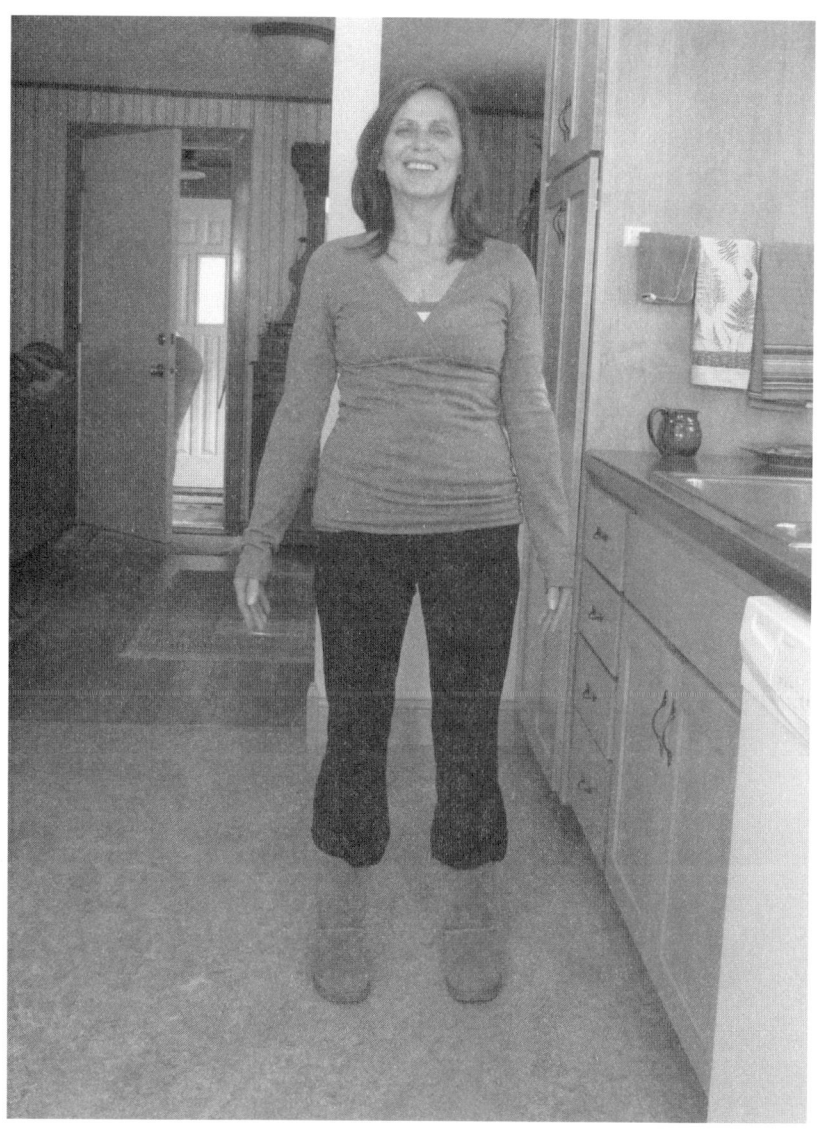

in the Kitchen

Standing Hamstring Stretch

You can do this anywhere there is a chair or low stool. Not everyone wants to do the hamstring stretch in bed, but tight hamstrings are *really* bad for our backs, so try to do a hamstring stretch regularly.

Stand up straight in front of your (preferably, cushioned) stool or chair and rest your heel on the seat. That, by itself, may give you a bit of stretch. If you're not feeling much stretch (or the sensation of stretching diminishes) you can go a bit farther. Keep your body straight from hips to head and bend forward from your hip just to the point where you begin to feel a stretch at the back of the thigh or knee of the leg that's resting on the chair. Hold the position and breathe deeply. Repeat with the other leg.

in the Kitchen

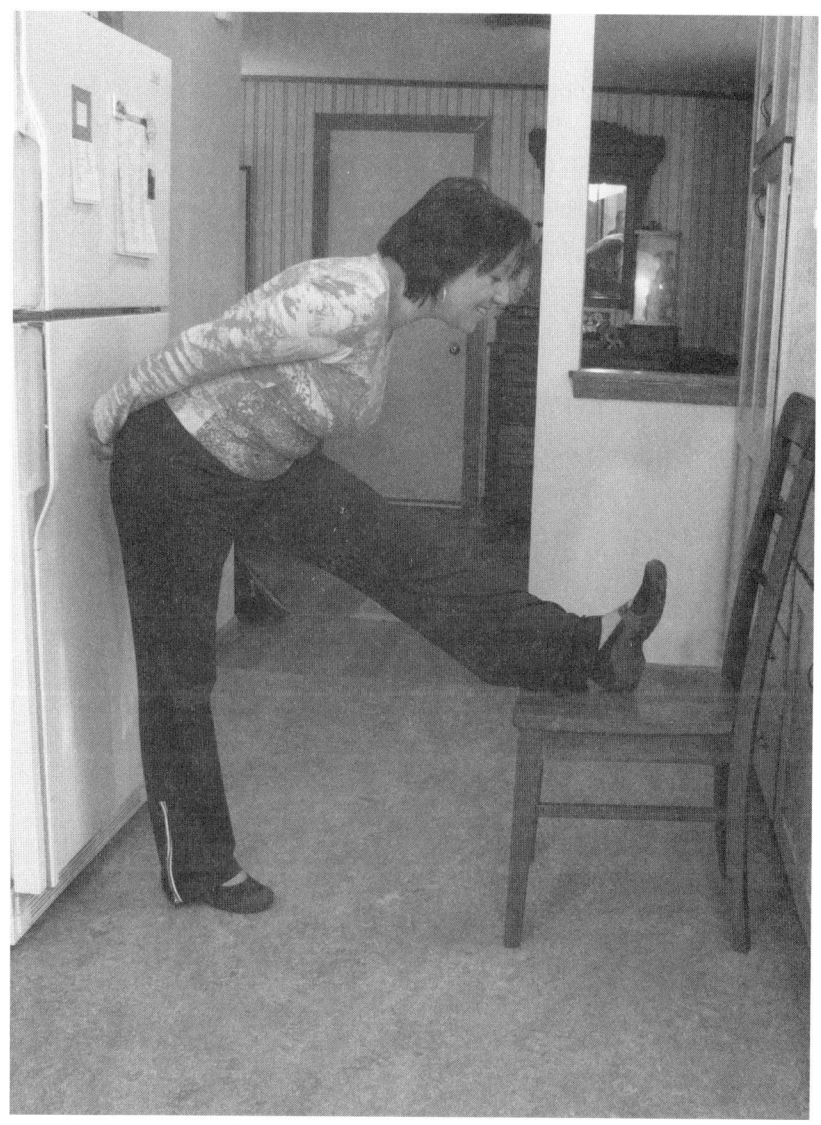

in the Kitchen

Palm Tree

Balance poses are a good barometer for how balanced you are in your life. If you feel centered and strong, balance poses will be easier for you than if you are kept off balance by crises. Balance poses can help you center and bring yourself into balance while improving your concentration. They also strengthen and tone leg muscles.

The palm tree is particularly good for strengthening feet and ankles, which will make all of the other balance poses ever so much easier (eventually).

Begin with the feet together and arms relaxed at your sides. As you inhale lift your arms out to the sides and over your head (keeping the backs of the hands facing each other) and at the same time rise up on your toes. Keep in mind that at first this will be a bit wobbly, but as the feet strengthen you will feel more solid. Hold the pose as long as possible (caramelizing sugar and family crises always taking precedence). It's fine if you need to lower your heels, then go back up again.

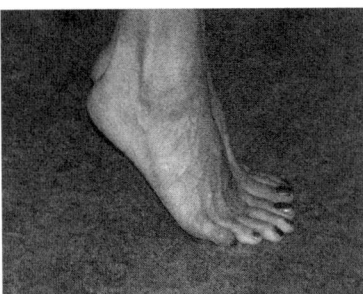

Not everyone needs to get their heels up this high.

in the Kitchen

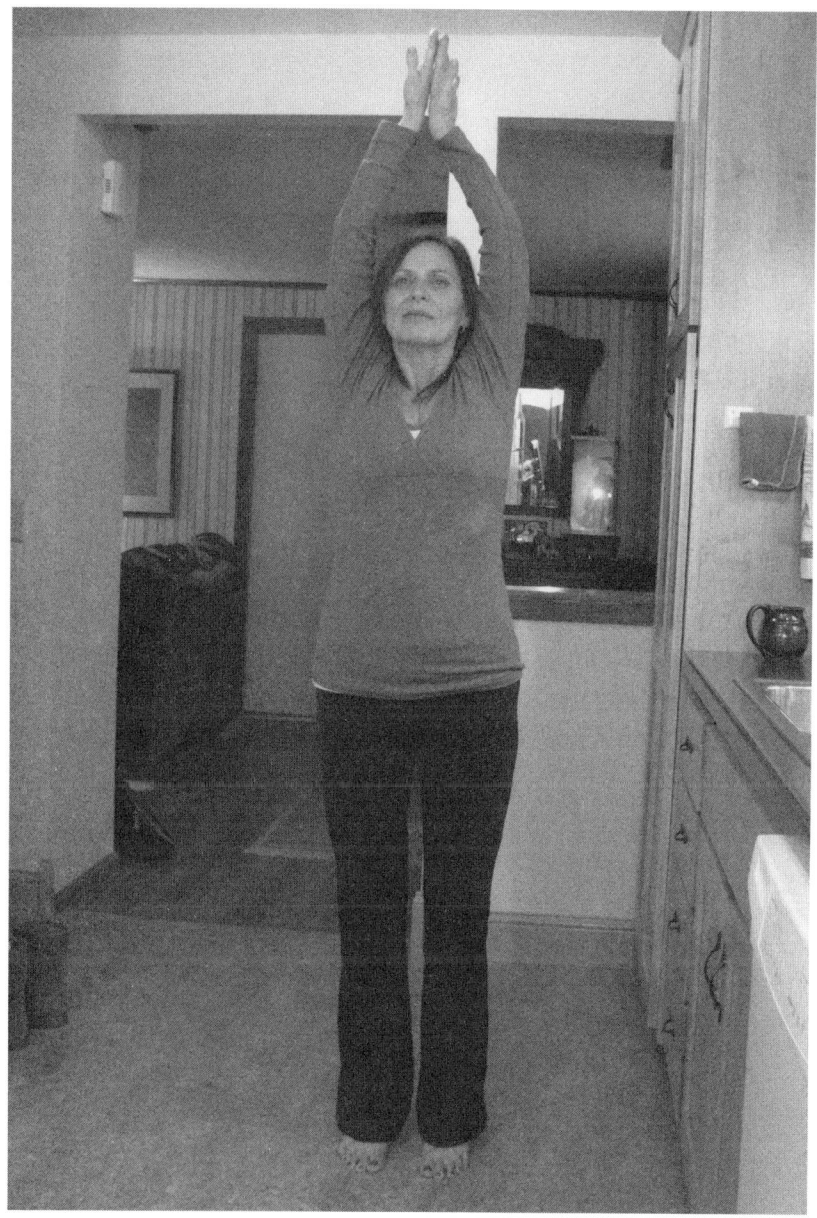

in the Kitchen

Pine Tree (My Name for It)

This is a classic balance pose. Start from a solid mountain pose. That is, feet shoulder width apart and hands at your sides relaxed.

To move into the pine tree pose, shift your weight over onto one foot. Turn the other foot out 90° and draw it back toward the weight-bearing foot. Lift the foot until it rests against your ankle (if your balance is poor), calf, knee, or thigh (if your flexibility and balance are good). If this is easy for you, you can rest your foot on the front of your thigh as high up as it will go without pulling your body out of vertical alignment.

Take a deep, slow breath and bring your hands together, finger tips touching and palms facing one another, in front of your heart. This is a mudra (hand position) that helps balance the energies of the body. It supports this balance pose and helps you concentrate. You can also bring your hands together over your head.

Repeat while standing on the other leg.

in the Kitchen

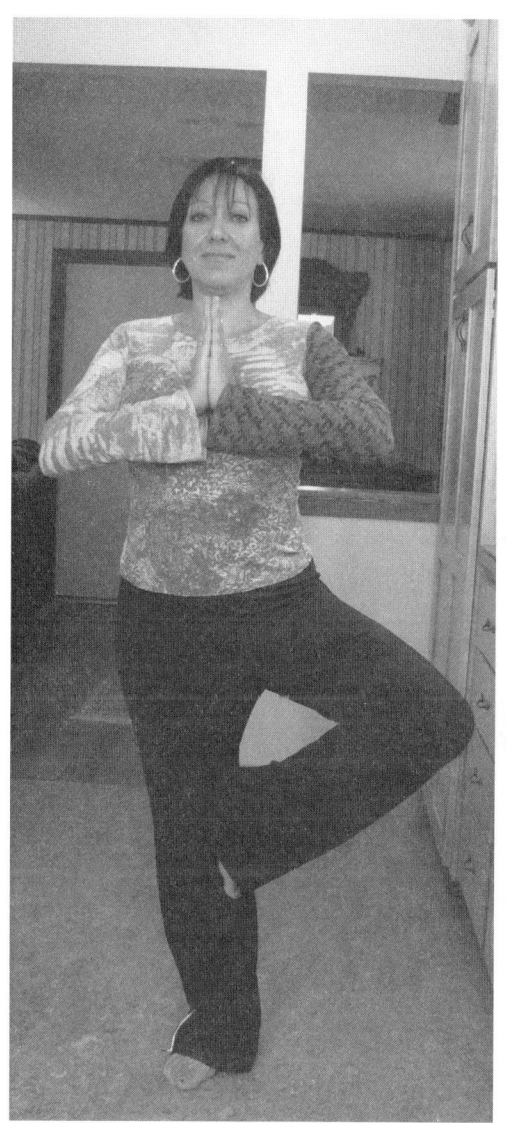
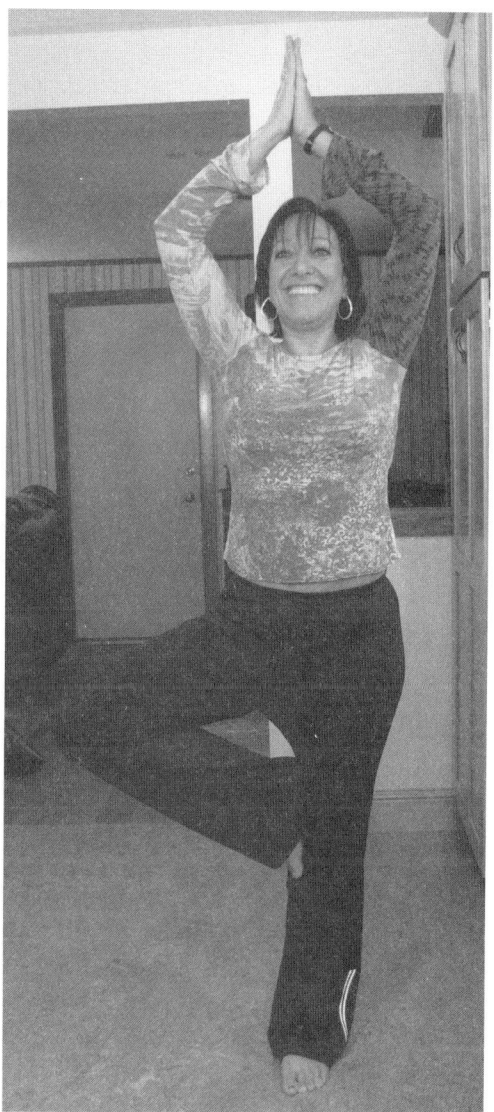

in the Kitchen

Kitchen Warrior I

The warrior poses seem to me to be about *owning* our space in the universe. In a yoga class, with everyone doing it together, it may not seem that way, but in a kitchen, with the spatula in one hand and the hotpad in the other, you can really feel the power of the pose.

Before you start, make sure your feet aren't going to slip. Either barefoot or with non-skid shoes on, begin in the mountain pose. Spread your legs as far apart as they will go without threatening pain or splitting your pants (if your pants threaten to give way, wear something knit next time). Turn your right foot out 90°. Turn your left foot in 45° *(see illustration below)*. Turn your body (from the hips on up) toward the right foot. As you inhale, lift your arms out to the side, parallel to the floor. Lift your arms straight up over your head and look up. Bend your right knee so that the shin is perpendicular to the floor. Take deep, full breaths.

If you feel you can use a little enhancement to the pose, imagine angels are holding your hands and pulling you upward. Feel the upward stretch.

Return to the point where your legs are spread but feet are pointed forward and repeat this pose to the left. Kitchen Warrior I opens your chest for improved breathing, as well as strengthening your legs, knees and ankles. It also improves balance and concentration.

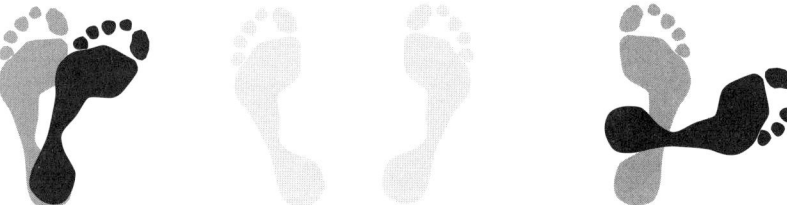

To get your feet into the warrior stance, begin with the lightest footprint and move to the darkest.

in the Kitchen

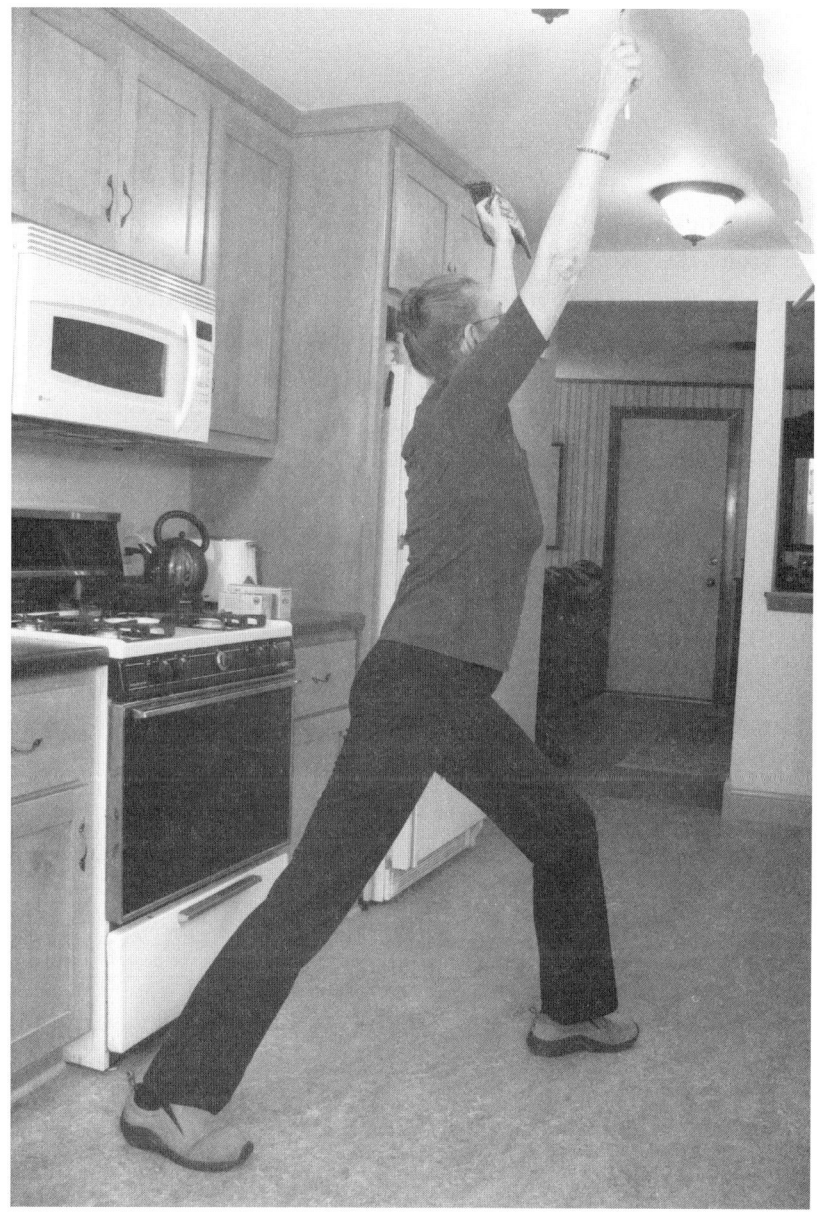

in the Kitchen

Kitchen Warrior II

Beginning in the same spread leg position as in Kitchen Warrior I, again turn the right foot 90° to the front and the left foot 45° in the same direction. *(See the illustration on page 70.)* Bend your right knee so your shin is perpendicular to the floor. Again, lift your arms until they are parallel to the floor and out to the side. Keep your body facing forward and turn your head to the right. Hold the position while you take several deep breaths.

Now, repeat this pose to the left.

This exercise has similar benefits to Kitchen Warrior I, with less opening of the chest. Instead, it encourages flexibility in the hips, since the body faces forward.

in the Kitchen

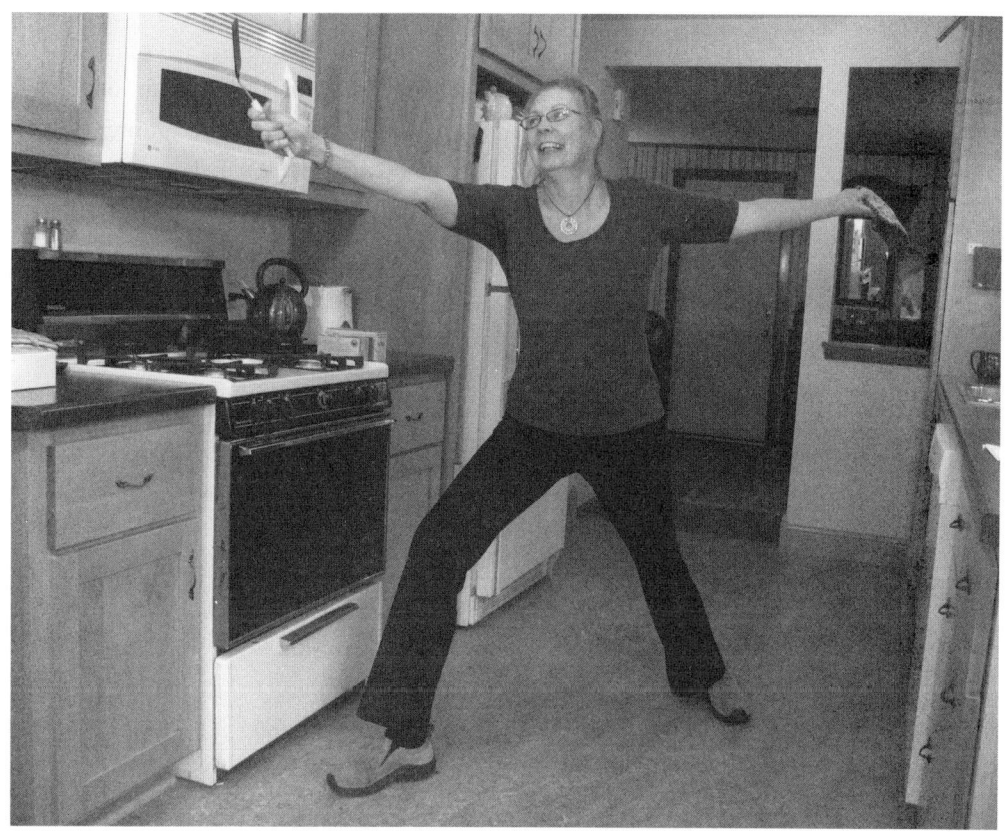

in the Kitchen

Supported Forward Bend

Facing the kitchen counter, place your hands on its edge with the fingers pointing away from you. Walk backwards away from the counter (leaving your hands in place) until your body is as near parallel to the floor as possible and your legs are vertical. Now, with your torso supported by your hips and hands, let it relax toward the floor. Hold this position for several deep breaths. Ultimately, you want your back to be concave in this position. Not everyone can achieve that right away. That's okay. There are still benefits to be had.

To come out of this pose, maintain a firm grip on the counter as you exhale and press your shoulders and spine up toward the ceiling. Hold that position for a few breaths, then step toward the counter and inhale as you stand up.

This pose opens the shoulders, stretches the back and counteracts the perennial slump that some of us have picked up over the years. It also stretches the hips. As mentioned in the section on yoga in bed, forward bends are about surrender, letting go of what you can't control, and about giving up the control freak persona.

in the Kitchen

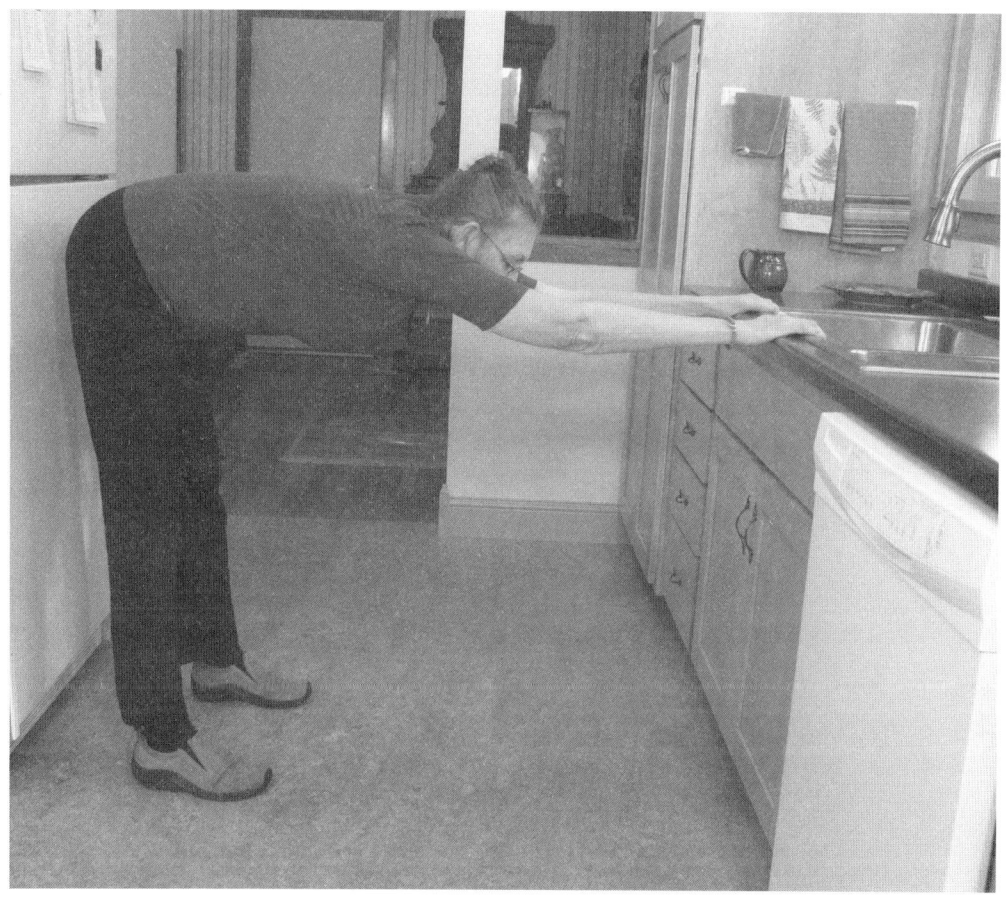

in the Kitchen

Backbend

If you do any kind of forward bend, you need to balance it with a backbend.

The easiest way to do this is to stand with your feet shoulder width apart. Place your hands on your hips with the fingers supporting your back. Inhale as you lift your chest and arch your back. Hold this position for several deep breaths.

This pose opens the chest, strengthens the abdominal muscles and stretches the front of the hips. Metaphysically, backbends are about trust (as mentioned in the section on yoga in the bedroom). Trust is something a lot of us have trouble with, so be gentle with yourself.

in the Kitchen

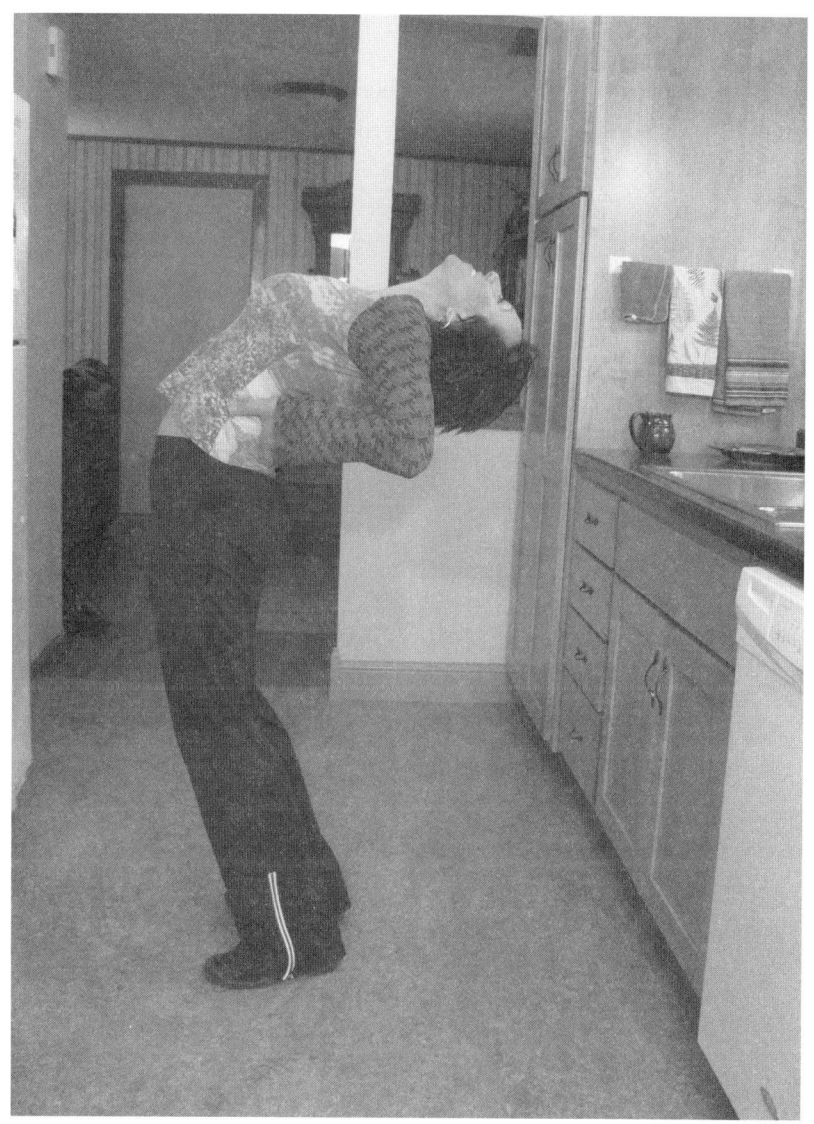

in the Kitchen

Plank at the Counter, Table or Chair Seat

This is a strengthening pose for back, belly, arms and upper body. It helps develop a thing called core strength. Core strength is vital to a healthy, stable back.

Begin by standing facing the counter. With your hands resting on the edge of the counter (or table or chair), take two or three steps back until you are leaning against it. Bringing your body into a straight line from shoulders to heels, breathe deeply and slowly. The position may remind you of the starting position for push-ups. Hold this position long enough to feel you've done something—or until the phone rings, whichever comes first.

As you grow stronger, you can choose lower and lower support for your hands: table, chair and, eventually, the floor. The trick is learning to feel when your body is in a straight line from shoulders to heels—like a plank. Ask the kids! They'll tell you.

in the Kitchen

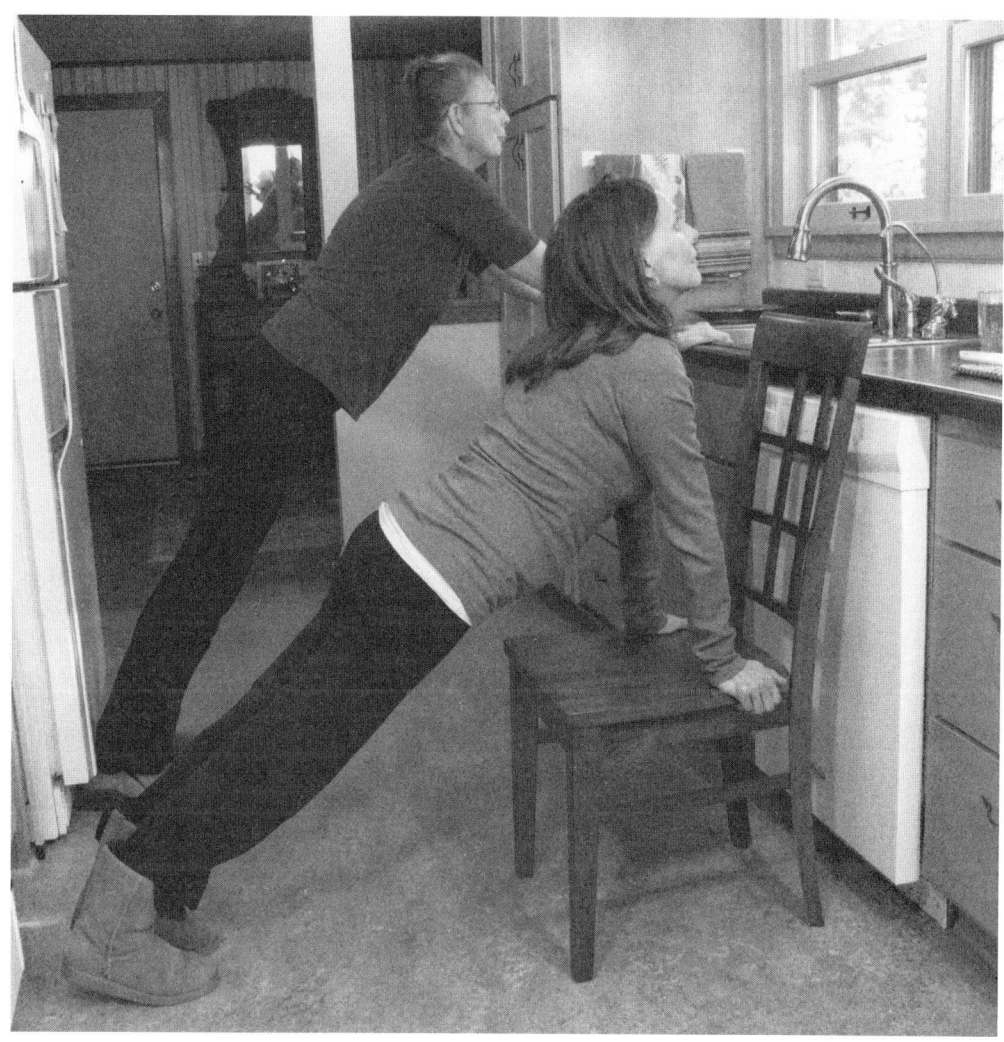

in the Kitchen

Dog in a Chair

Downward Facing Dog is one of yoga's classic poses. It also can be rather challenging. This variation provides a way to get many of the benefits while building the strength and flexibility required for the classic version.

Place the back of a kitchen chair against a counter, wall, or something else that won't go anywhere, with the seat facing you. Bend down so you can grasp the sides of the seat with your hands. Step backward until you begin to feel a stretch in your Achilles tendon. Take another step back as you bend forward from your hips, lowering your shoulders and head until your head is between your arms and your body is in a straight line from hands to hips. Press your hips toward the ceiling. Imagine your position as an upside down "V".

As you take a deep breath, imagine that the breath goes directly to wherever you feel the stretch. As you exhale that breath, imagine your body relaxing into the pose. Let your shoulders release toward the floor. Take several deep, slow breaths before stepping back to the chair and standing up.

Not only does this exercise strengthen and stretch, it provides some of the benefits of inversion poses like the shoulder stand, or head stand. It clears the head, opens the chest, stimulates the immune system, and reverses the effects of gravity on the body (thus slowing, and, sometimes, reversing the aging process).

in the Kitchen

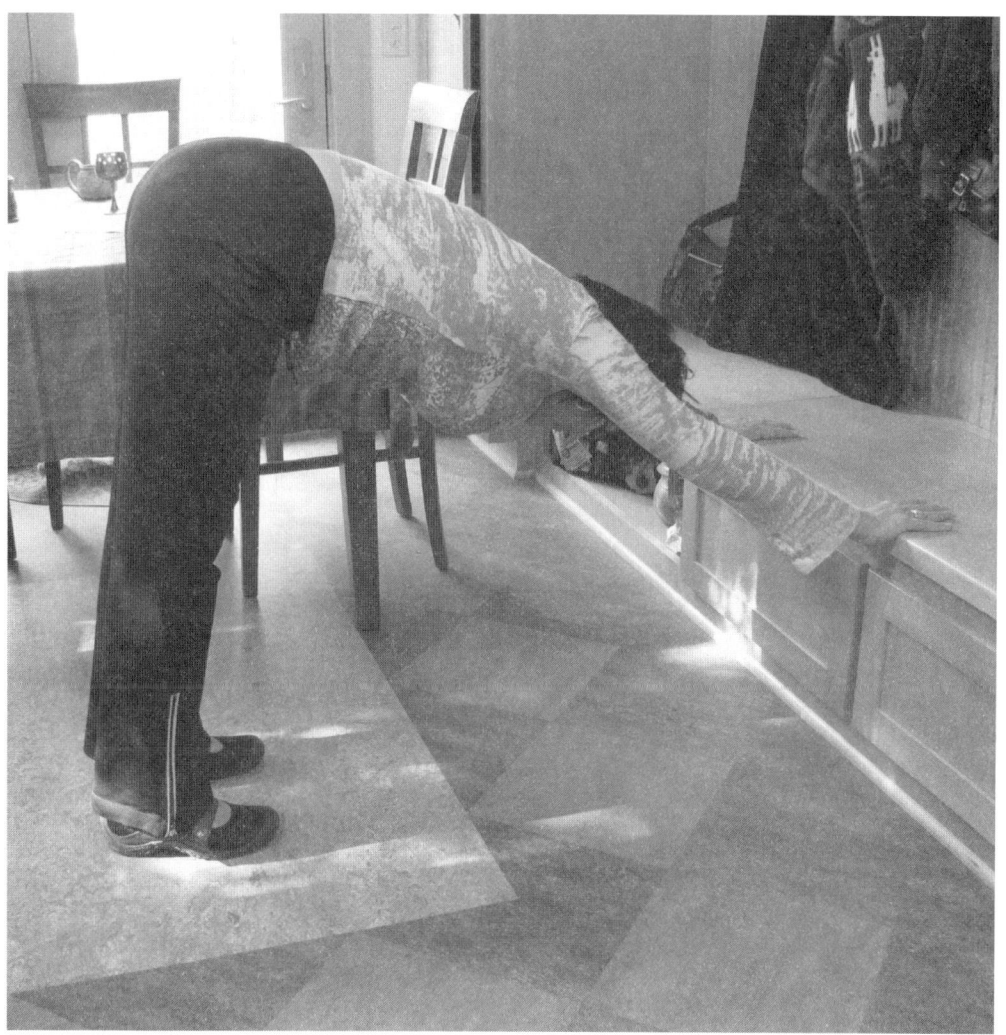

in the Kitchen

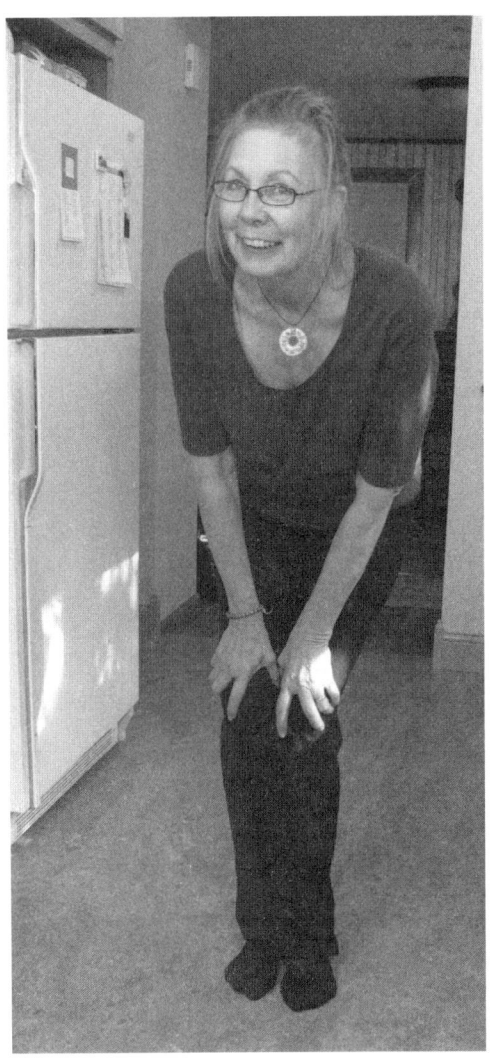

Knee Circles (or Knee Chi)

This exercise both strengthens and increases flexibility in the knees. If you've got a taste for dancing the jitterbug, this will help you there too.

With feet and knees together, bend your knees slightly and rest your hands just above them, thumb to the inside, fingers to the outside. Rotate both knees to the right three or four times and then to the left the same number of times.

Inhale and stand back up.

Spread your feet so they are shoulder width apart. Bend your knees and rest your hands just above them, thumb to the inside, fingers to the outside. Now rotate them out and away from one another three or four times. Reverse direction and rotate them toward one another three or four times.

Inhale and stand back up.

in the Kitchen

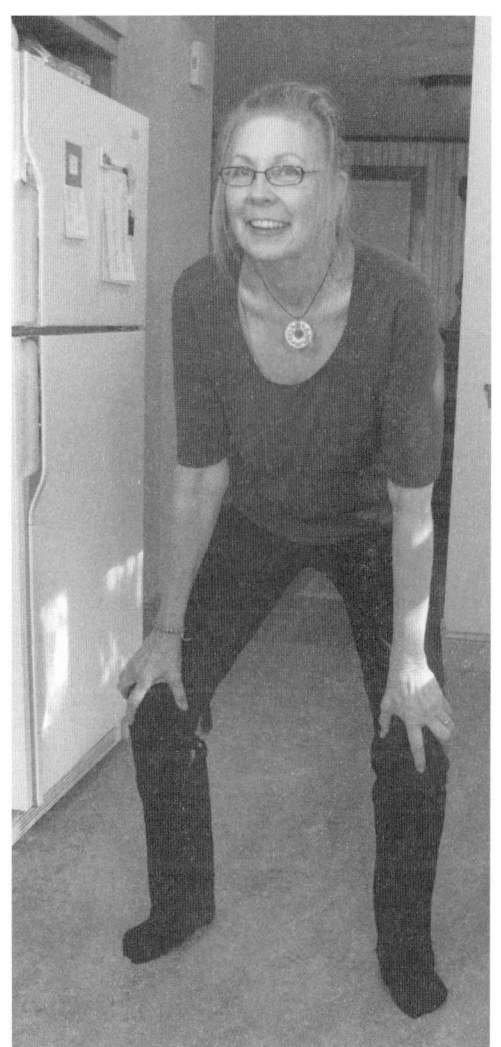
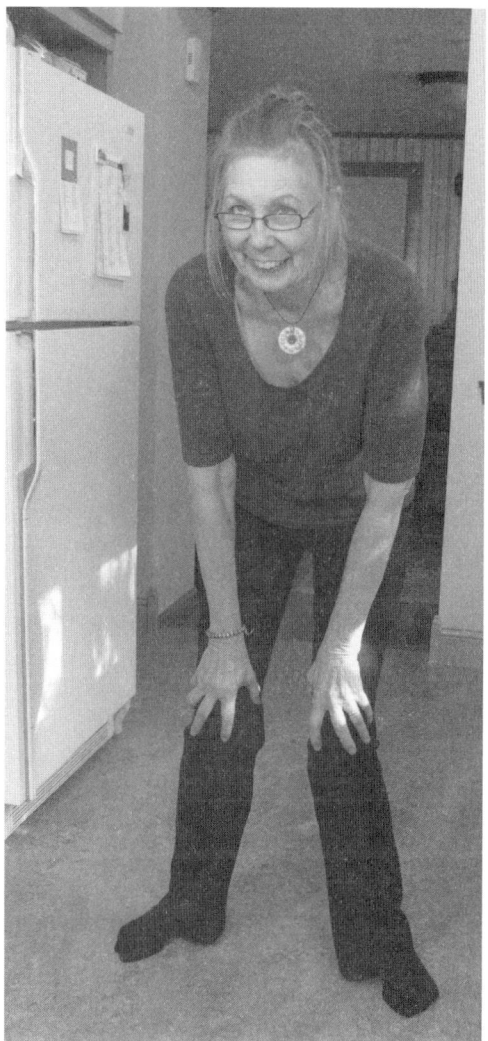

in the Kitchen

Do You Have a Dining Room?

Use some of the poses from the kitchen and check out poses from Office Yoga and Bedroom Yoga. There are even poses from Sofa Yoga you can do at your dining room table, providing your guests are game or you're dining in solitary splendor!

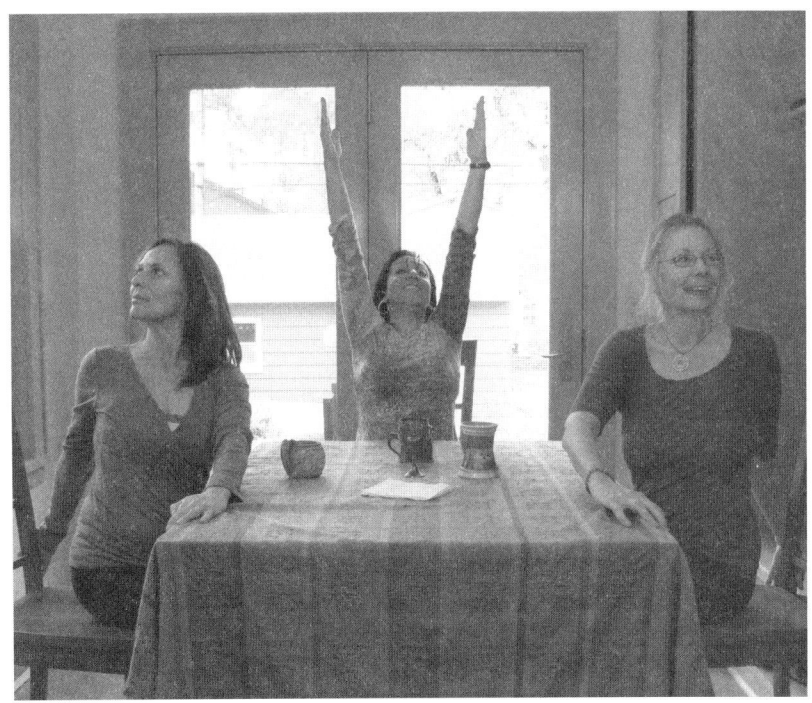

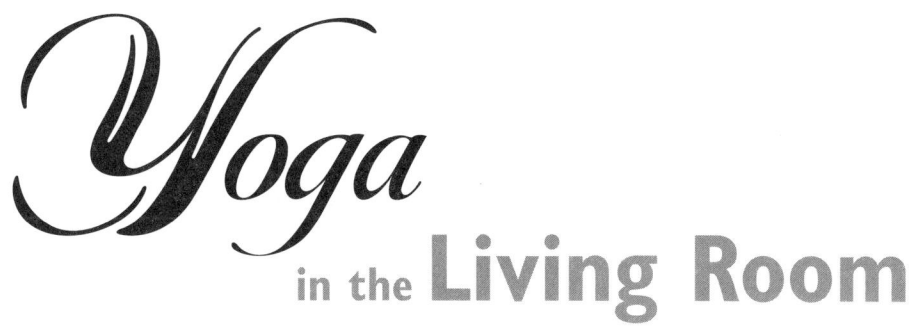
Yoga in the Living Room

So, you're watching TV. That doesn't mean you can't do yoga. The sofa is a great place to do some stretching.

in the Living Room

Fingers, Hands and Wrists

This series is particularly important for people who spend a lot of time in front of computer screens or at cash registers, because they are probably spending way too much time tapping keys or pushing a mouse around. These activities jam fingers and bring on repetitive motion problems like carpal tunnel syndrome.

1. With your arms stretched out in front of you, spread your fingers as far apart as they will go. Hold that stretch for two or three breaths. Next, make a tight fist keeping your thumb on the outside, wrapped around the fingers. Hold for two or three breaths. Repeat the stretch and fist at least three times.

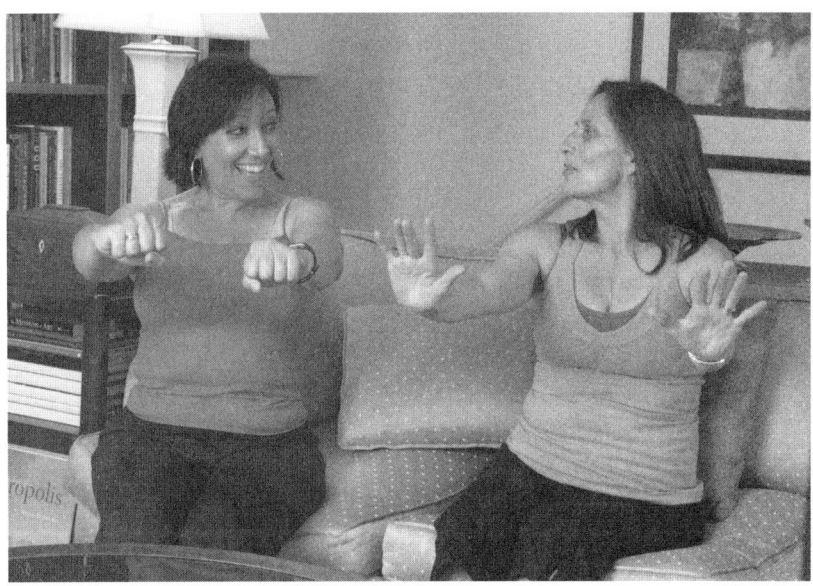

in the **Living Room**

2. Begin again with your arms stretched out straight in front of you. This time palms face out and fingers are together pointing up. Keep your hands parallel to one another (as best you can) as you rotate them around your wrists. Palms out as you swipe them across the top arc. When your palms are horizontal, flip them over so your palms are facing you. Sweep them across the lower arc and when your palms are horizontal with the fingers pointing in the opposite direction, flip your hands over again so the palms are facing outward again. Do three or four complete circles in one direction before reversing directions and doing three or four revolutions in the other direction. Relax your hands and shake them.

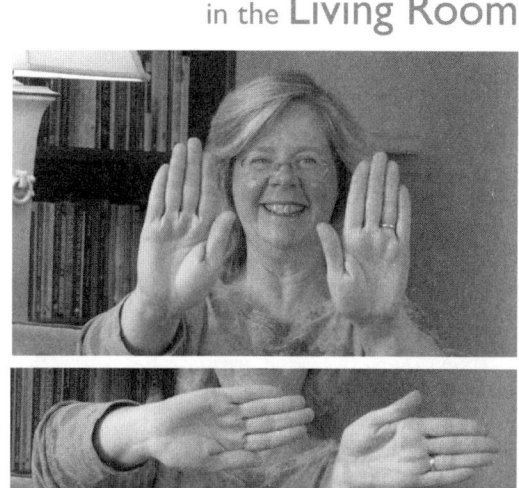
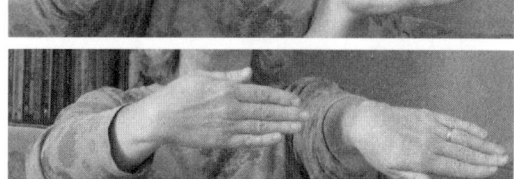
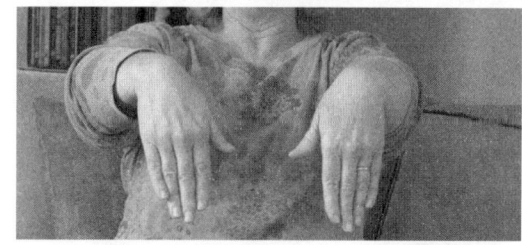
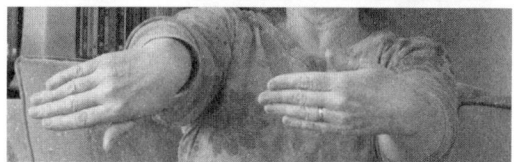
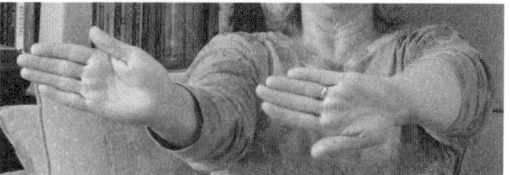

in the Living Room

3. Sit up straight (don't worry, it's only for a few moments) and bend your left elbow so your left forearm is parallel to the floor across the front of your body. Bend your wrist so that your fingers are pointing skyward. With your right hand, push gently back on the fingers to gently stretch your fingers and wrist. Keep the forearm parallel to the floor. Hold the position and breathe into the stretch. Release.

Next, with the same arm parallel to the floor, bend your wrist so the fingers and hand are pointing toward the earth. Use the right hand to push on the back of your left hand gently toward the bottom of your forearm. Keep the forearm parallel to the floor. Hold the position and breathe into the stretch. Release. Repeat both operations on the right hand.

in the Living Room

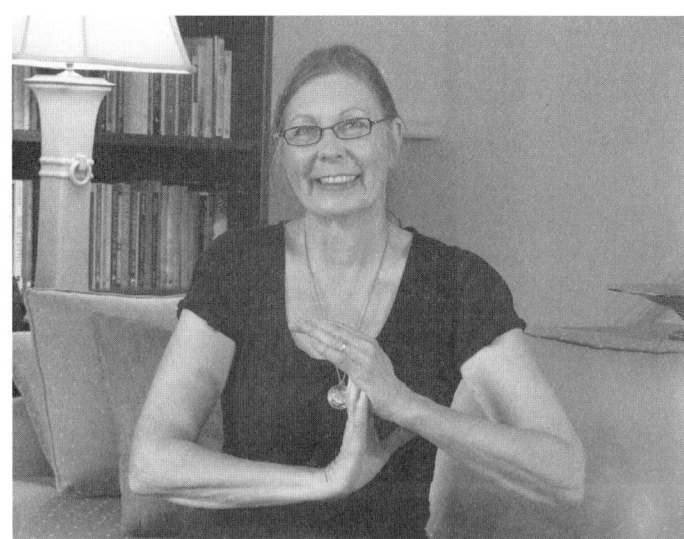

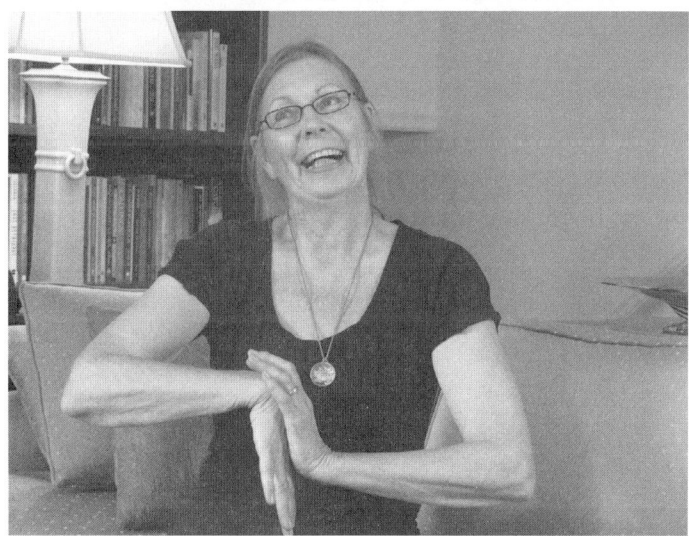

in the Living Room

Toes and Feet

Our feet are our foundation in the world. They also get almost no attention or respect in our daily lives. Many women's feet, in particular, are pulled from their natural healthy state by the shoes they wear. Now's the time to change that!

1. Sit up straight, resting your right ankle on your left knee. Interlace the fingers of your left hand with the toes of your right foot. Make sure the fingers go in as far as they can (preferably all the way up to the palm) and as close to the base of the toes as possible. If your toes are too tightly packed to allow your fingers in, grab a handful of pens or pencils to spread the toes apart. You could also get those cushy toe-spreaders used for painting toenails.

Breathe several deep breaths, remove the fingers (or other spacers) and repeat with the left foot.

The rest of these exercises can be done while slouching if you so desire!

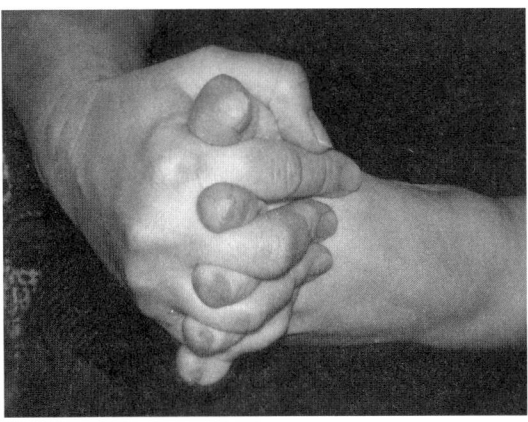
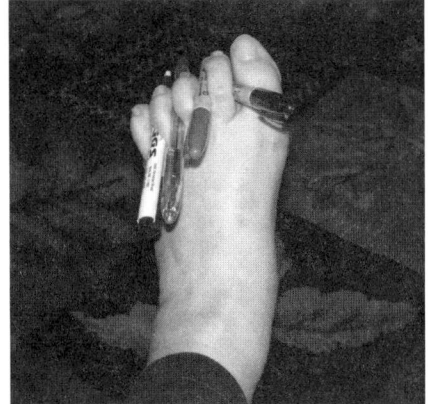

in the **Living Room**

2. Spread your toes as far apart as they will go—really stretch them. Take a full, deep breath. Now, roll your toes up tight like a fist (no need to try to wrap the big one around the others—after all, we can't *really* make a fist with our feet). Take a full, deep breath. Stretch your toes and clench them at least twice more. Relax.

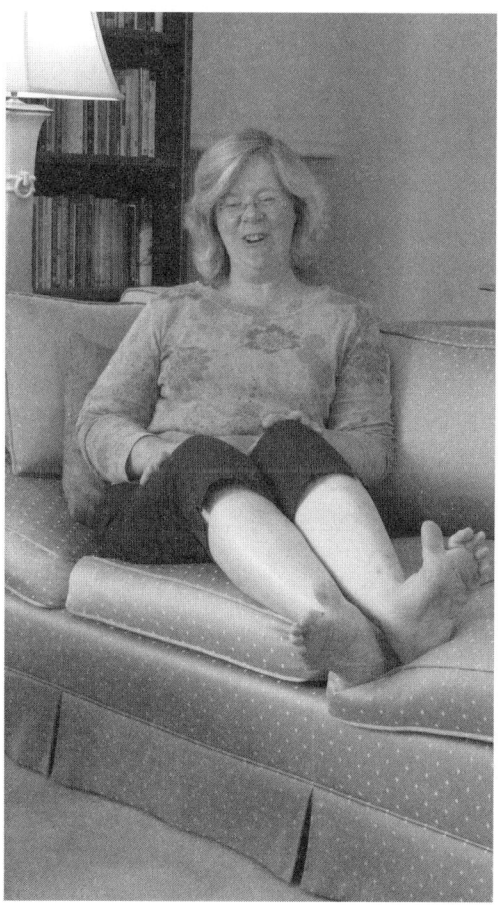 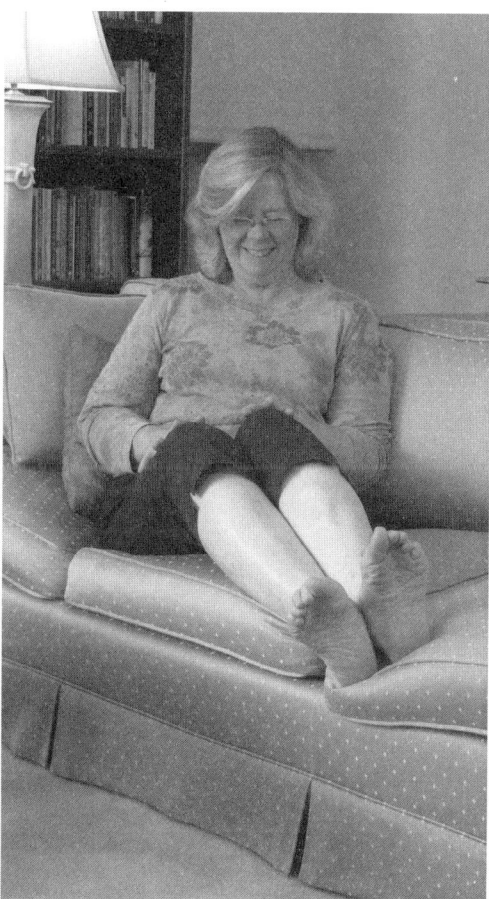

in the Living Room

3. Keeping your feet as parallel to one another as possible, do three or four ankle circles in each direction. As time goes on, increase the number of repetitions.

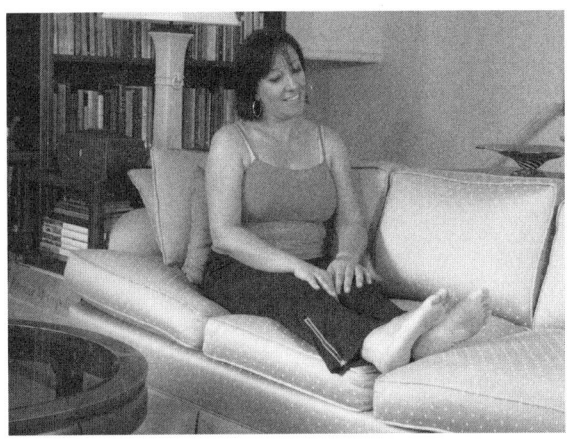

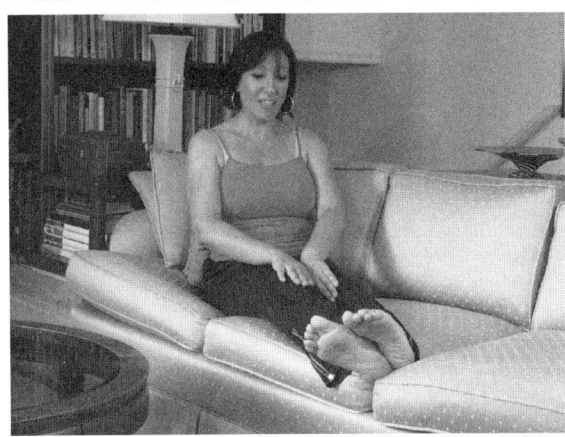

in the Living Room

4. Bend your ankles so that your toes are pointing up towards your knee and you feel the stretch in your Achilles tendon. Hold that position for a breath. Point your toes toward the opposite wall. Hold that position for a breath. Alternate these stretches three or four times and as time goes on you can increase the number of repetitions.

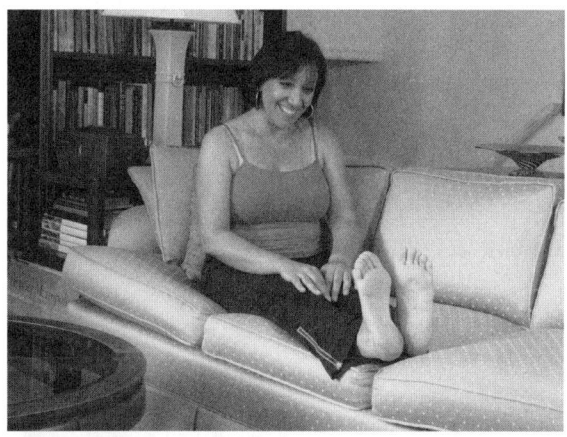

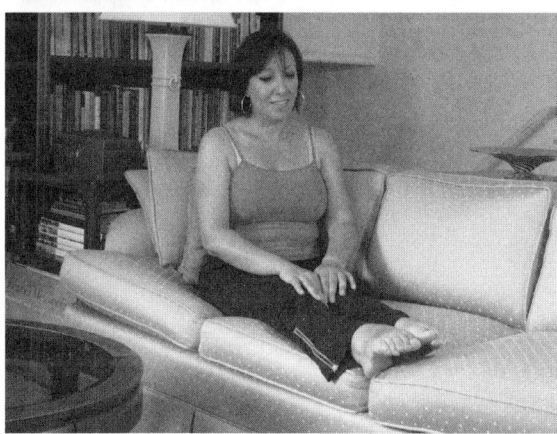

in the Living Room

Scaring the Cat

Give your face some exercise and stretching. Keep the facial muscles youthful and toned. All you need to do is squeeze your entire face in tight around your nose. Hold for several seconds.

Now, act really surprised. Draw your eyebrows up to your hairline and open your eyes as wide as they will go. Open your mouth until your lips stretch (make sure they're well moisturized first) and pull your jaw toward your chest. So, maybe your eyebrows won't merge with your hair and your jaw won't hit your chest without bending your neck. It's the intention that counts.

Alternate these positions several times while reading or watching your favorite show. Try not to do it in front of your kids' friends. It'll scar your kids for life.

in the Living Room

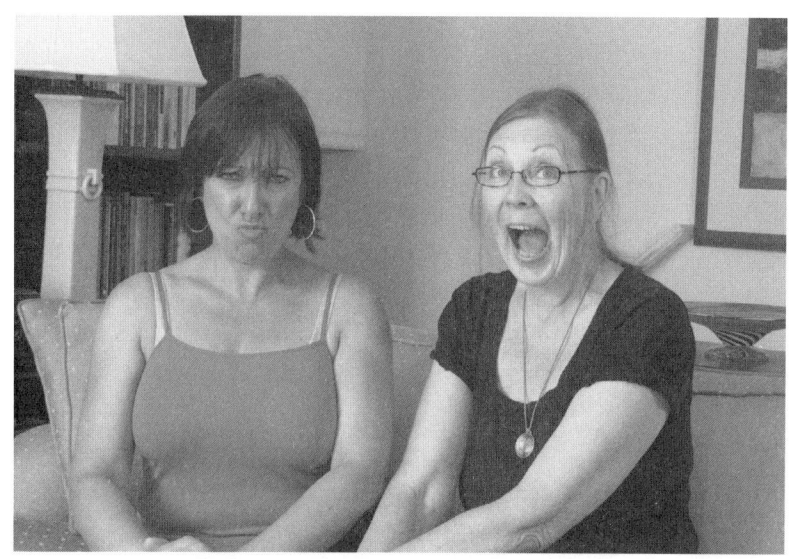

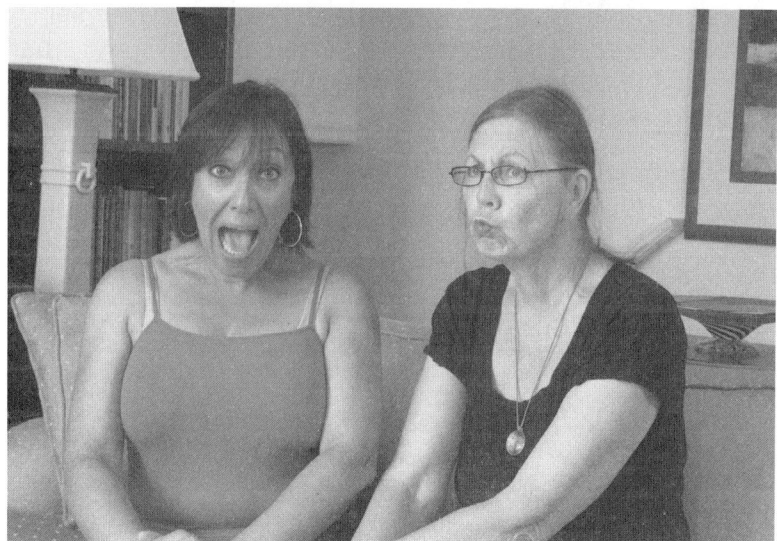

in the Living Room

Lion Pose

Here's another great one for embarrassing the kids if they're older. If they're younger, they may well want to join you. You can be a pride of lions! Combining yoga and play you can boost everyone's immune system and fight off any little bugs that are trying to get a foothold. If the TV's on with something everyone wants to watch, do this during commercials. It is definitely distracting.

Sitting toward the front edge of the sofa or chair, or kneeling on the floor with your hands resting on your knees, take a *deep* breath. Fill your lungs right up.

Here's the tricky part. As you expel *all* the breath in your lungs in a great and sudden push (explosive even) you also: 1) Spring up from your sofa or heels with your hands outstretched (and all the fingers spread wide) as though you are pouncing on a hapless gazelle; 2) Stick your tongue out as far as it will go; 3) Open your eyes as far as they will open; and 4) Try to look at the spot on your forehead between your eyebrows.

Much laughter will ensue as you practice and practice while trying to remember everything at once. And the laughter is as good for you as anything!

in the Living Room

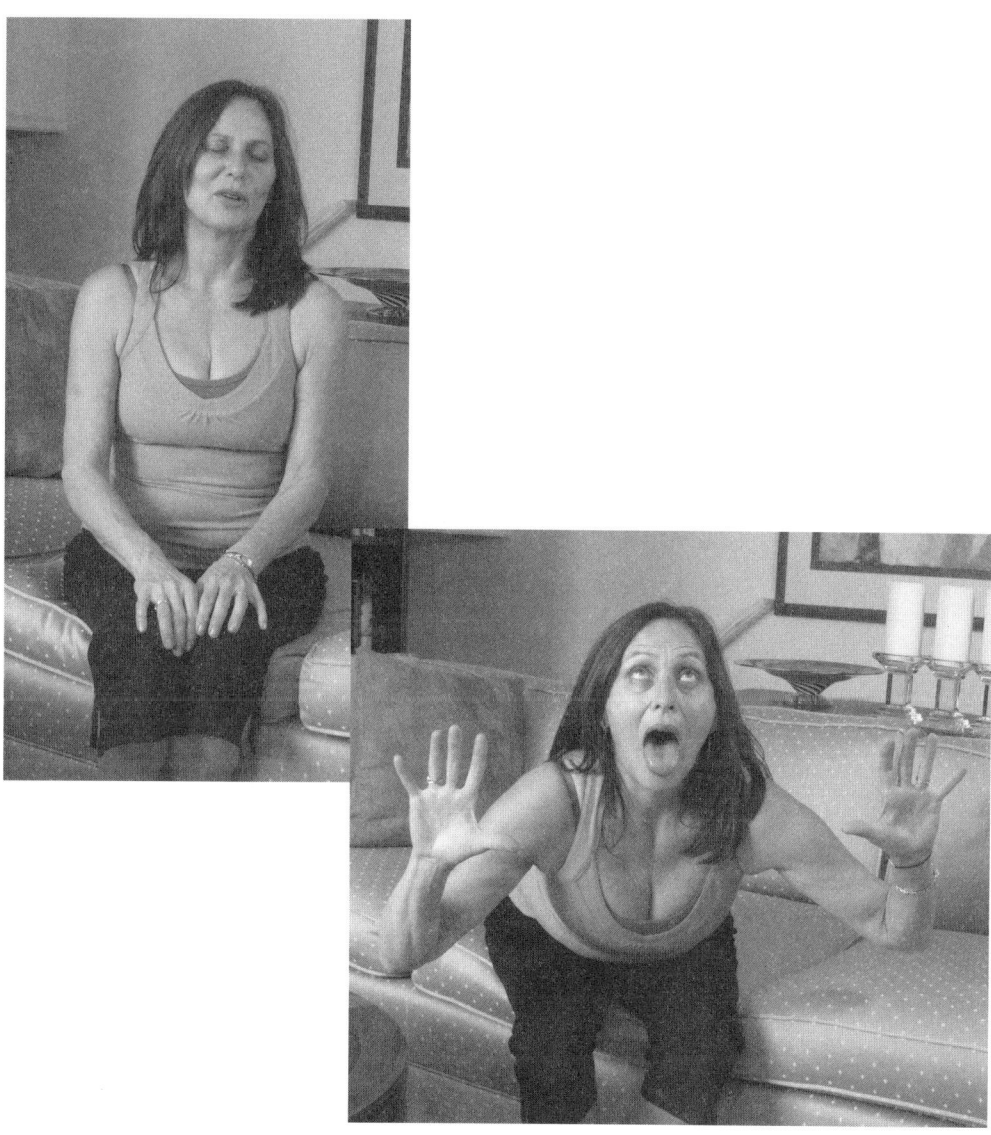

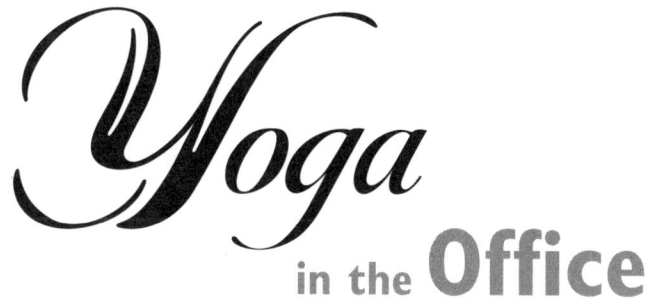
Yoga
in the Office

We start with a couple of exercises that are particularly useful in the office. Then we revisit some of the poses we talked about earlier, which will translate well to any office whether at home or at work.

in the Office

Angel Rescue Mission or "Reach for the Sky, Pardner!"

You've been sitting in one position for way too long. It's time to reclaim your right to erect posture. But you have to go a little beyond mere standing up to get back in balance.

Stand with your feet about shoulder width apart. As you inhale, raise your arms out to your sides and continue that motion until your fingertips are pointed at the ceiling. Imagine angels have grabbed your hands and are trying to lift you up to heaven, but you're just not ready. Or, imagine you're on the roof of a house in the midst of a raging flood and really good-looking rescuers are trying to lift you into the helicopter. The idea is that you feel the stretch all along the length of your body.

Stretch upward for three or four deep breaths, then clasp your hands together and, rotating around your waist, imagine you are drawing circles on the ceiling. Make three or four circles in one direction, then three or four in the other direction.

Release your hands and let them float lightly down to your sides.

Are you feeling better?

PS: This pose can be done from a sitting position if standing would cause too much disruption, or if standing is not on your menu.

in the Office

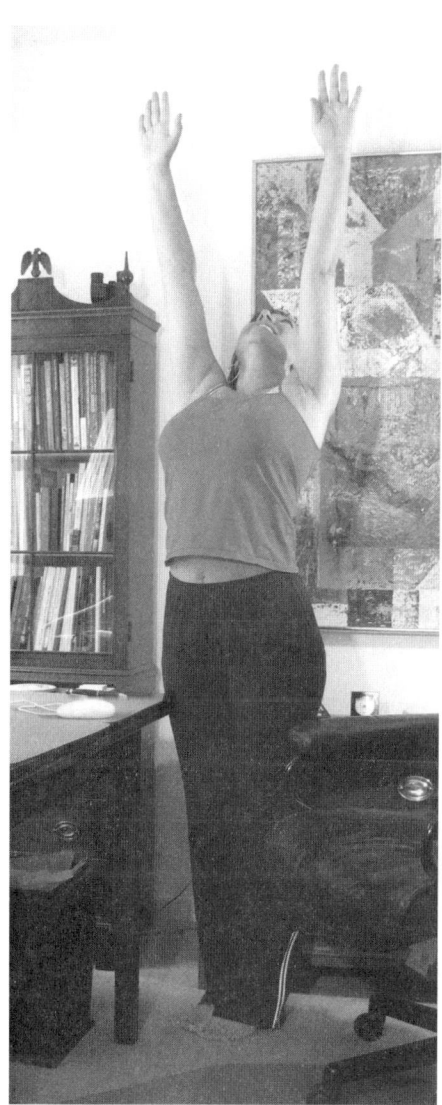
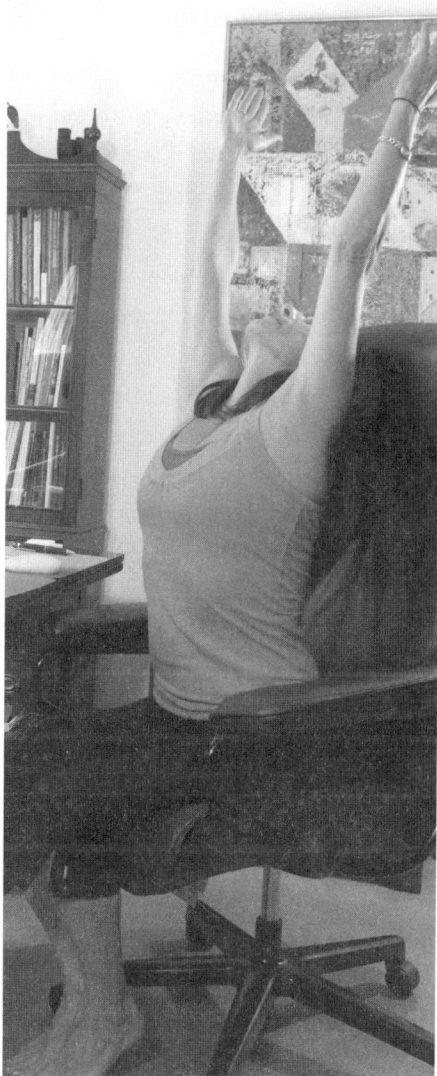

in the Office

Reversing Gravity: The Shoulder Stand

You may want to find a bit of privacy (and some open floor space) for this one. I have never found a replacement for the good, old-fashioned shoulder stand. If you are doing this at work maybe you could enlist a co-worker to guard the door (make sure it's not someone who will sell tickets).

If this pose seems a little too physically challenging, skip down to the next exercise. Same benefits, less effort. You may still want the guard at the door.

Why do either one? Being upside down for a few minutes (even one) will clear your head (at least for a while) whether you're just not thinking clearly or you have a head cold. It also reverses the effects of gravity on the body and stimulates the immune system.

For comfort's sake, you may want to place a thinly folded blanket or a folded jacket under your shoulders—*not* under your neck.

Begin by lying down on the floor (jacket beneath your shoulders, guard at the door), bend your knees and rock back onto your shoulders until your hips and legs are over your head. Brace your body by propping your hips up with your hands. Don't worry about how straight your body is. It's more important for there to be no strain on your neck. Breathe.

Hold this position for as long as you feel okay about it, up to three minutes. Roll down gently.

Counter this inversion by arching your back and allowing your head to hang back for a few breaths. I recommend that you also massage your lower back by lying on the floor, pulling your knees up to your chest and rocking back and forth and side to side.

You will be far more capable when you get back to work!

in the Office

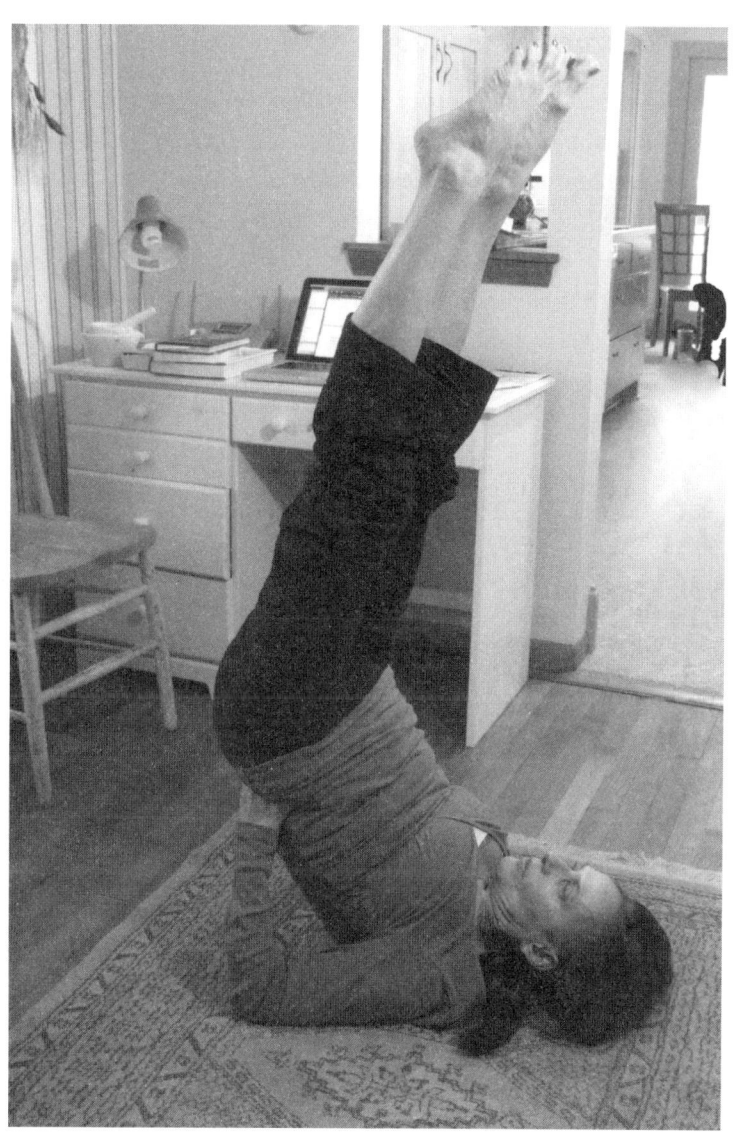

in the Office

The Shoulder Stand Made Easy

If your chair is braced against a wall or heavy desk you can place your feet against the front of the chair seat and press your hips up into the air for a while. Brace your hips with your hands and breathe deeply. You could also scooch your heinie up against a wall (or closed door) and bend your knees so that the soles rest flat against it. Push your hips up into the air as high as possible using your feet as leverage. Brace your hips with your hands and breathe deeply. Either from chair or wall, this does most of what the full-fledged shoulder stand does and is within pretty much everyone's capabilities.

in the Office

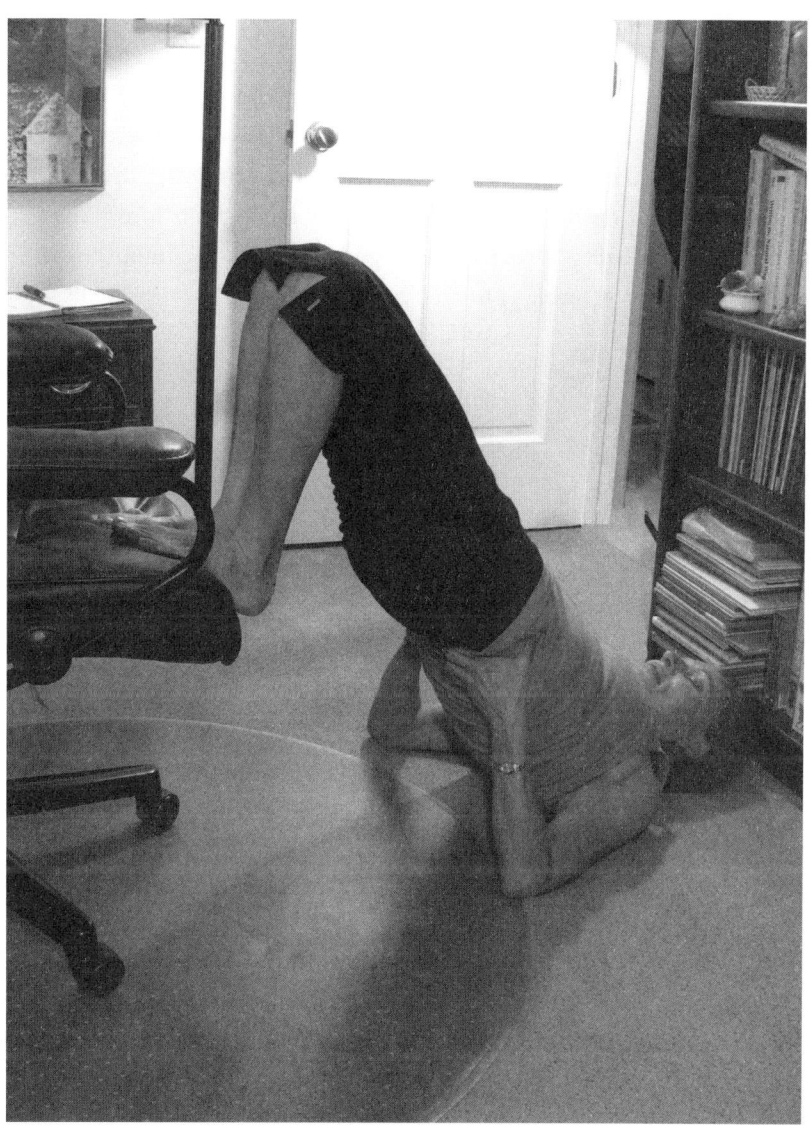

in the Office

Legs in Chair Pose

If the above poses are too scary, fear not! You can lie on the floor with your behind up against the front of a chair and rest your feet and calves in the chair. It may not be quite as effective for clearing your head, but it is relaxing and restorative. Do this for a few moments before going to that board meeting, after the meeting to restore your equilibrium, or after work before meeting your true love for dinner.

in the Office

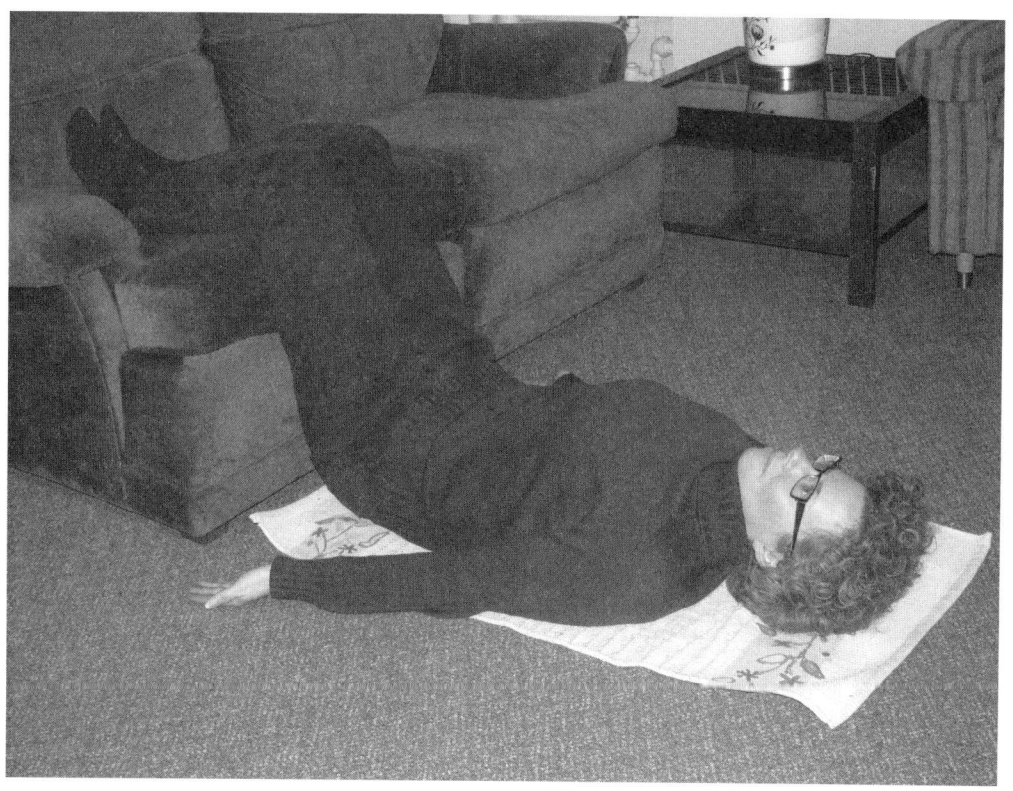

in the Office

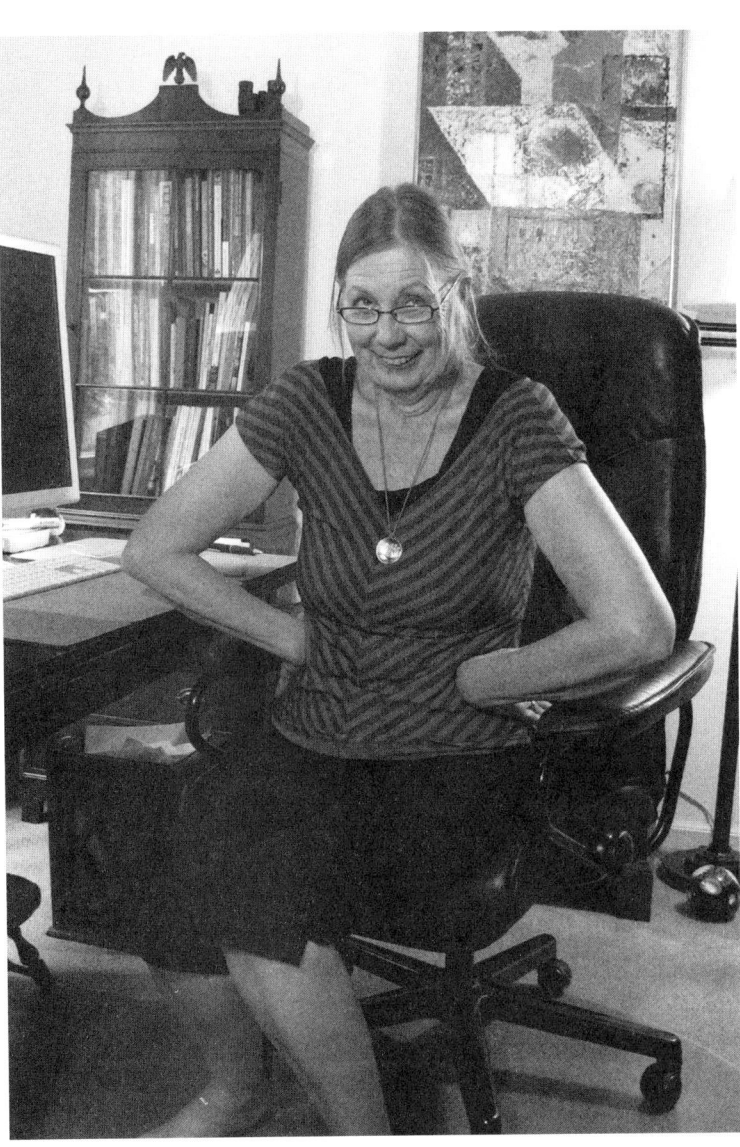

Torso Flip (or the Vertical Cat)

Maybe your pants are too tight to do a full-fledged forward bend. This will help. It may even rejuvenate you.

Sit upright toward the front of your chair, hands on your knees or hips. Inhaling, lift your chest toward the sky and drop your head back, pulling your shoulder blades together. Exhaling, lift your head, tuck it forward toward your chest, pull your shoulders forward and try to press your spine right through the back of your chair. Inhale and exhale as you flip back and forth several times.

in the Office

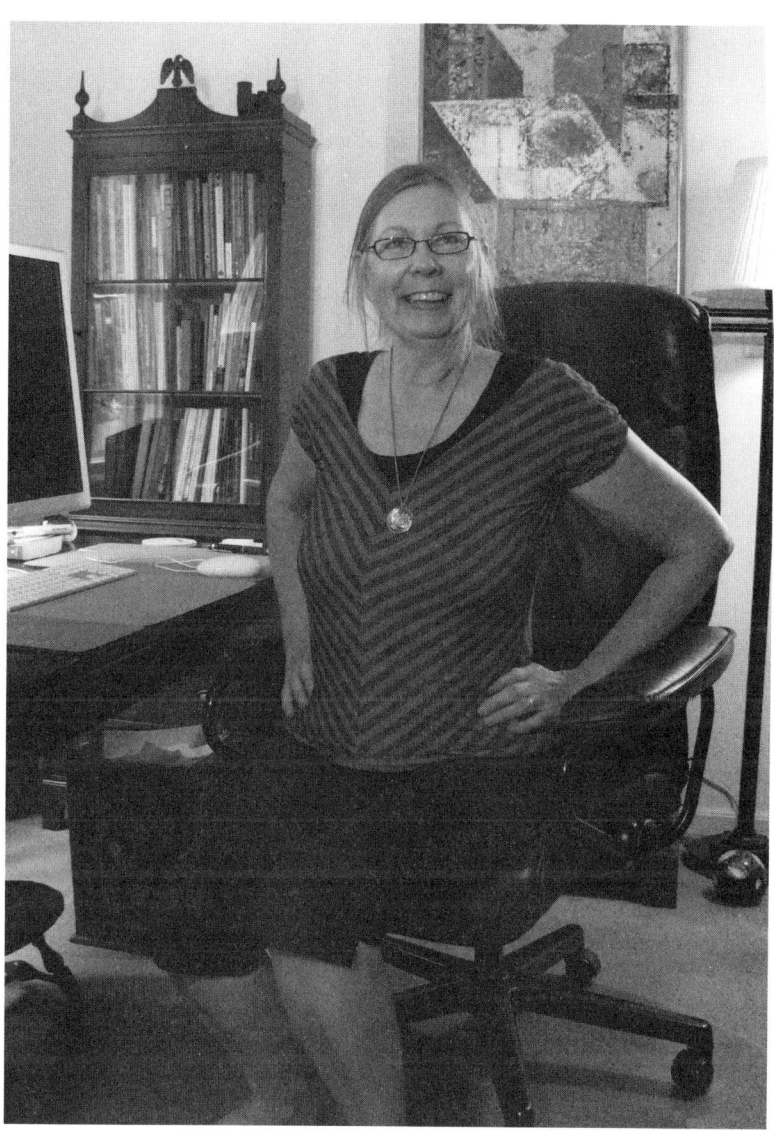

in the Office

Repeating the Good Stuff

You can bring several exercises we use in other rooms into the office. These are the ones I've found most useful when spending long periods of time in front of a computer screen.

Supported Forward Bend . . . Revisited

Stand facing your desk. Place your hands at its edge with the fingers pointing away from you. Walk backwards away from the desk (leaving your hands in place) until your body is as near parallel to the floor as possible and your legs are vertical. Now, with your torso supported by your hips and hands, let it relax toward the floor. Hold this position for several deep breaths.

To come out of this pose, maintain a firm grip on the desk as you exhale and press your shoulders and spine up toward the ceiling. Hold that position for a few breaths, then step toward the desk and inhale as you stand up.

This pose opens the shoulders, stretches the back and counteracts the perennial slump that deskwork can cultivate. It also stretches the hips.

in the Office

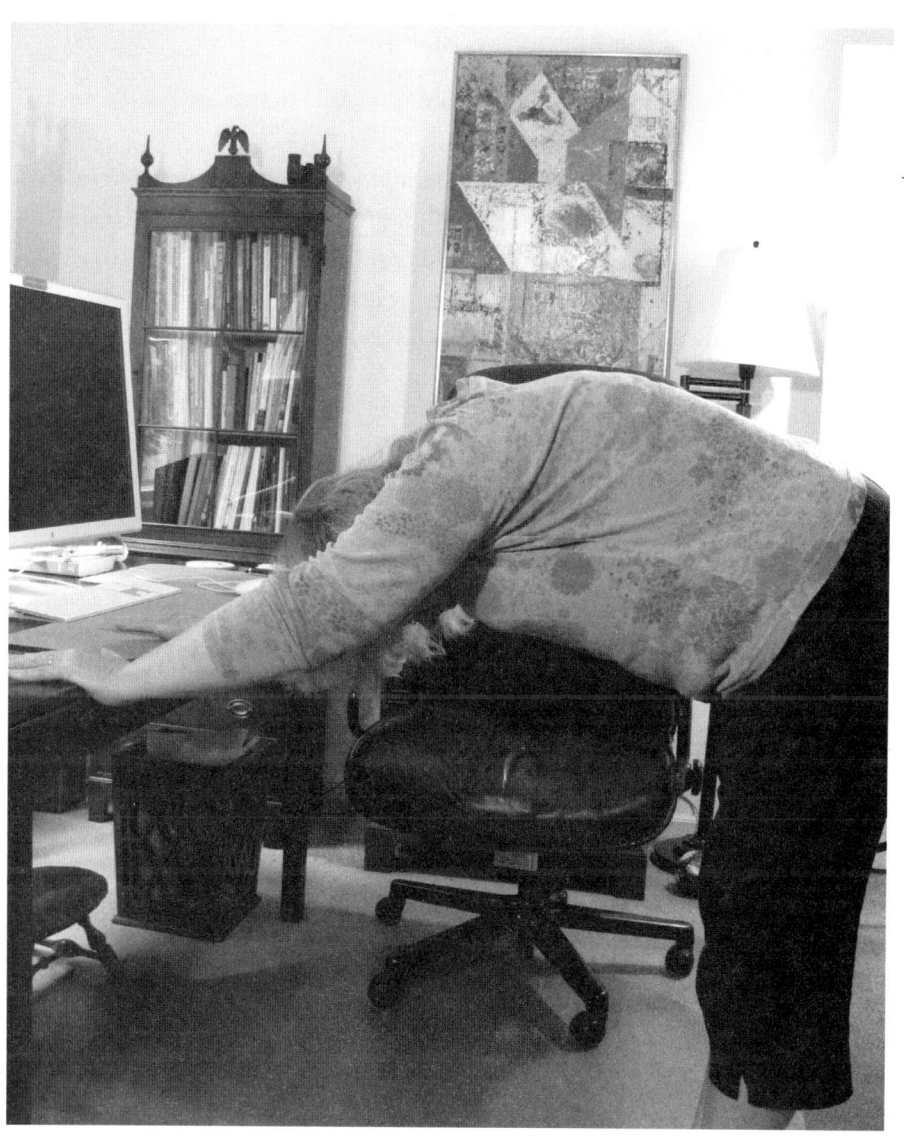

in the Office

Supported Backbend . . . Revisited

If you do any kind of forward bend, you need to balance it with a backbend.

The easiest way to do this is to stand with your feet shoulder width apart. Place your hands on your hips, preferably with the fingers supporting your back. Inhale as you lift your chest and arch your back. Hold this position for several deep breaths.

This pose opens the chest, strengthens the abdominal muscles and stretches the front of the hips.

in the Office

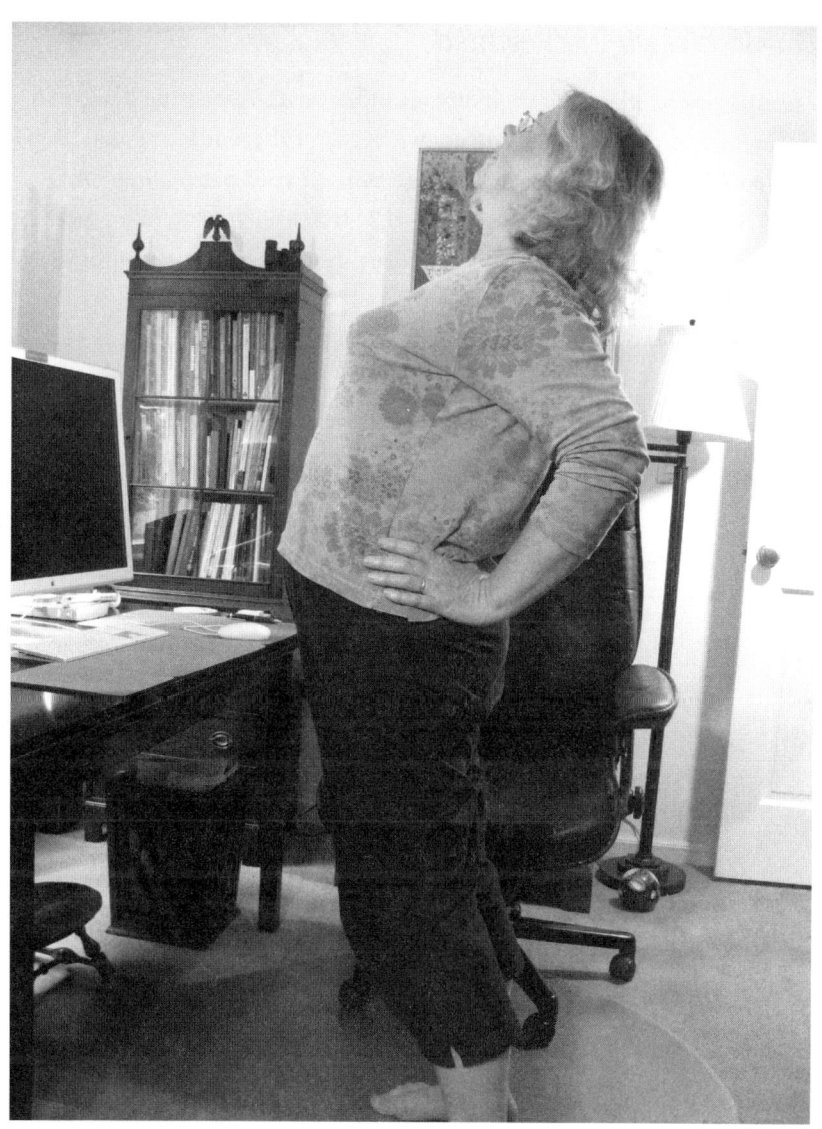

in the Office

Dog in a Chair . . . Revisited

For this classic, place the back of your office chair against the desk, wall or something else that won't go anywhere, with the seat facing you. Bend over so you can grasp the sides of the seat with your hands. Step backward a few steps until you begin to feel a stretch in your Achilles tendon. Take another step back as you lower your shoulders and head until your head is between your arms.

Imagine as you take a deep breath that the breath goes directly to wherever you feel the stretch. As you exhale that breath, imagine your body relaxing into the pose. Take several deep, slow breaths before stepping back up to the chair and standing up.

in the Office

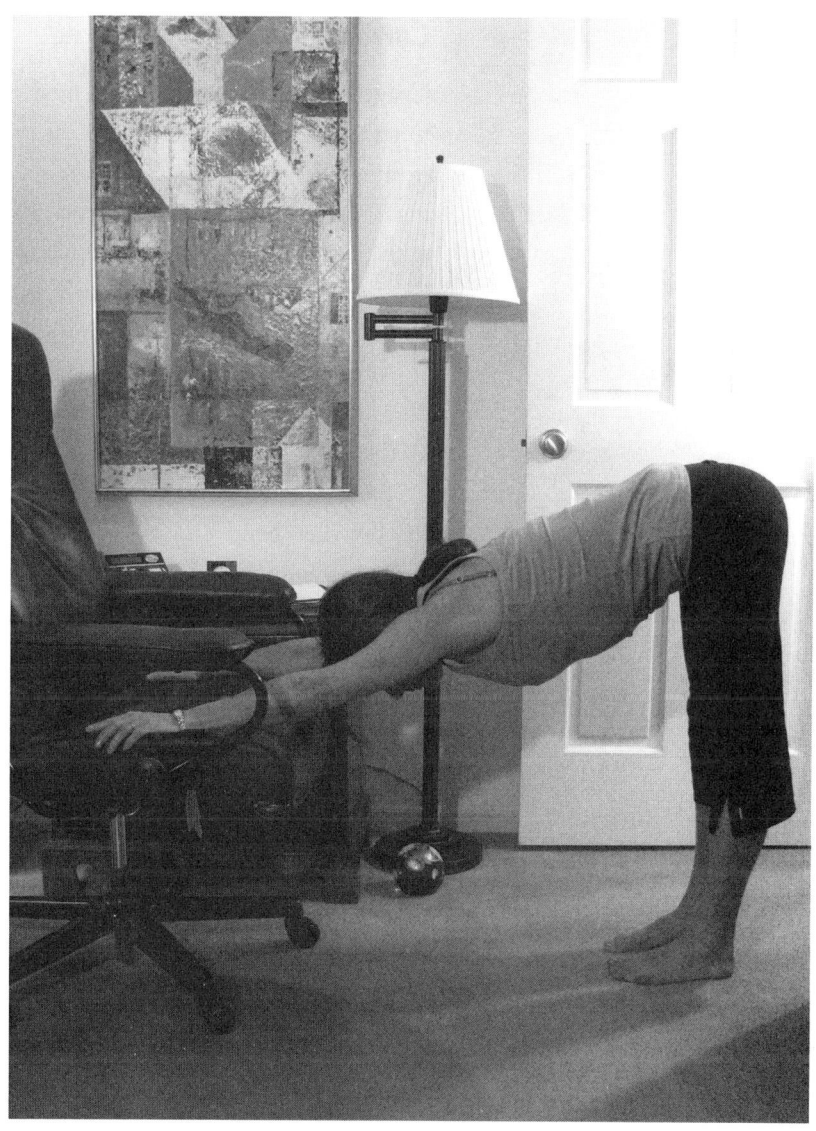

115

in the Office

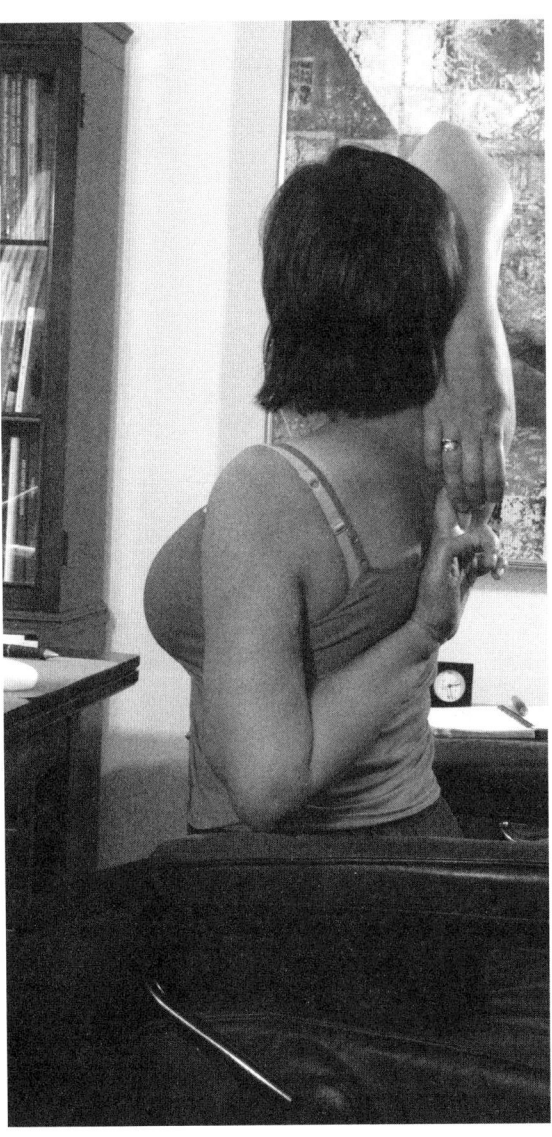

Cow Face Pose . . . Revisited

Crouching over the keyboard tends to encourage the muscles across the front of the chest to shorten, causing a hunched posture you carry with you everywhere. This habitual hunch makes you look older and less self-confident than you really are and spoils the look of your strapless ball gown. The Cow Face Pose counteracts all that.

Start by stretching one arm toward the sky, then bend your elbow so the forearm and hand dangle down behind the head. With the other hand reach behind your back and up until the hands meet and can clasp one another. If they don't reach, use a scarf or old tie to bridge the distance and work your hands as close together as possible.

Hold the position for a few breaths and switch sides.

in the Office

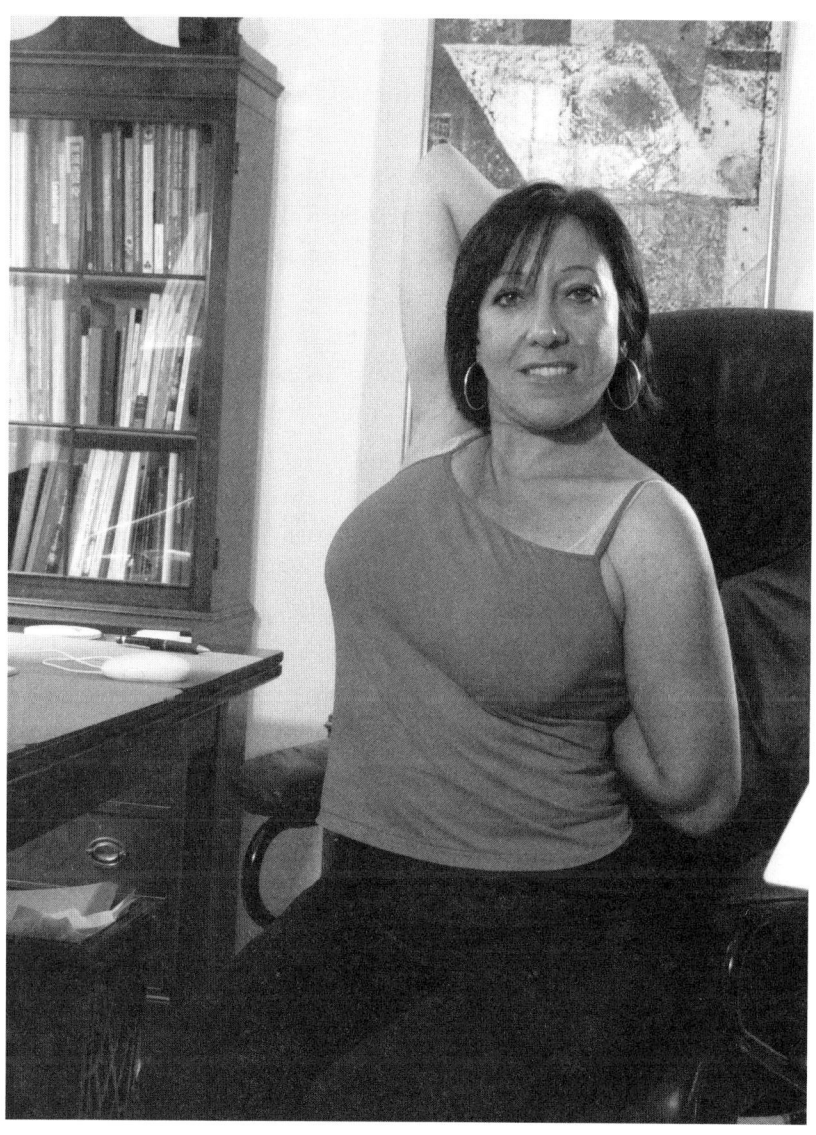

in the Office

Fingers, Hands and Wrists . . . Revisited

This series is particularly important to people who spend a lot of time in front of computer screens because they are often spending way too much time tapping computer keys. This activity jams fingers and brings on repetitive motion problems like carpal tunnel.

1. Hold your hands in front of you and spread your fingers as far apart as they will go. Hold that stretch for two or three breaths. Now, make a tight fist keeping your thumb on the outside wrapped around the fingers. Hold for two or three breaths. Repeat the stretch and fist at least three times.

2. Hold your arms stretched out straight in front of you, palms out, fingers pointing up. Keep your hands parallel to one another (as best you can) as you rotate them around your wrists. Do three or four complete circles in one direction before reversing directions and doing three or four revolutions in the other direction. Relax your hands and shake them. *(See pages 87 and 89 for illustrations.)*

3. Sitting up straight with the left forearm parallel to the floor, bend your wrist so that your hand is pointing skyward. With your right hand, push gently back on the palm to stretch your wrist. Keep the forearm parallel to the floor. Hold the position and breathe into the stretch. Release.

Next, with the same arm parallel to the floor, bend your wrist so the hand is pointing toward the earth. Again use the right hand to push it gently back toward your forearm. Keep the forearm parallel to the floor. Hold the position and breathe into the stretch. Release. Repeat both operations on the right hand.

in the Office

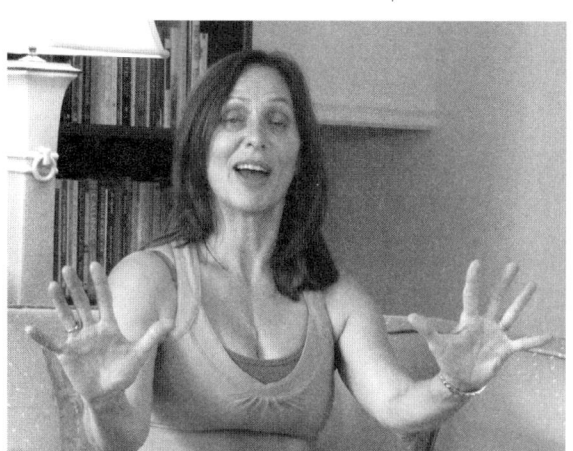
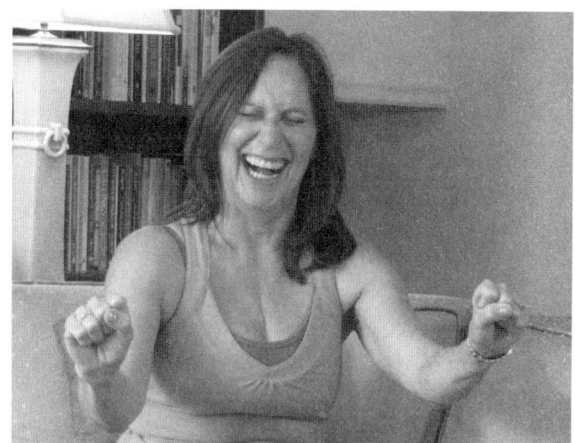
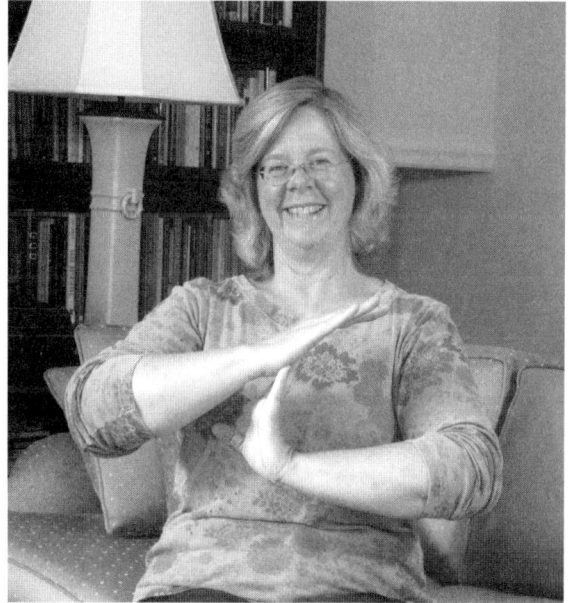
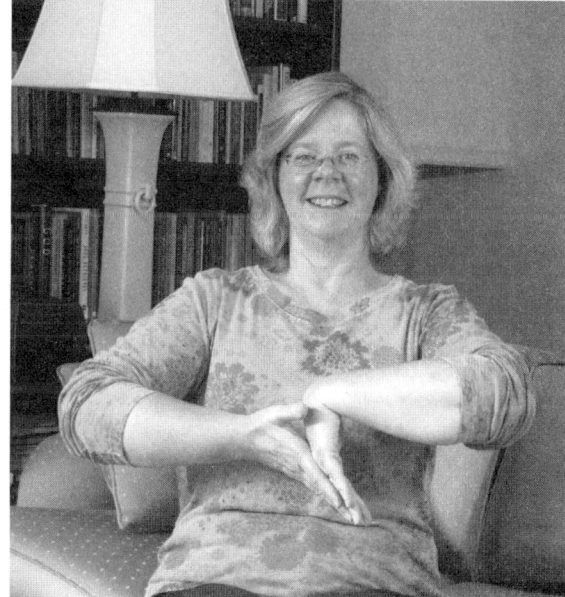

in the Office

Twisting, Turning . . . Revisited

This pose is great for a back that's been in the same position for too long. It also massages your internal organs and stimulates digestion (especially important given what you probably ate for lunch).

Seated on the edge of your chair, with your back straight, place your right hand on the outside of your left knee. Twist your body to the left as you reach behind with your left hand as far as you can reach and grab the back of the chair. Use your hands for leverage to help you twist even farther in that direction and turn your head as far around in the same direction as possible. Hold the position for two or three deep, full breaths and relax back to the front. Do the same thing in the opposite direction.

in the Office

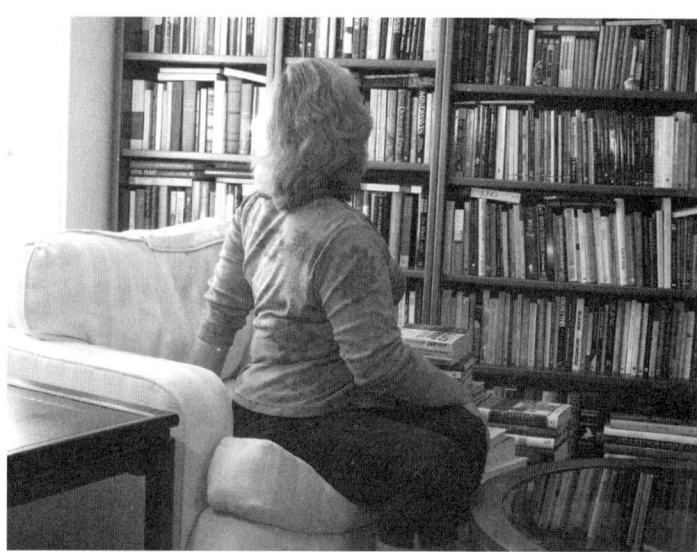

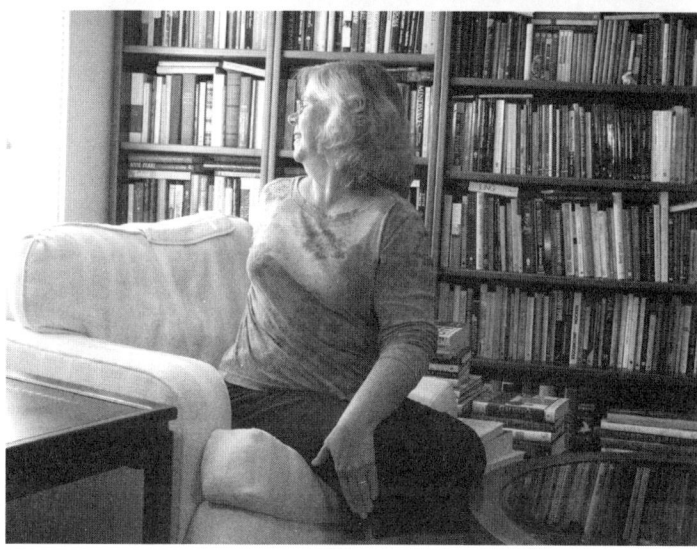

in the Office

Seated Forward Bend . . . Revisited

To do the seated forward bend in a chair, sit at the very front edge of your chair (only the sitting bones on the chair). Spread your knees far enough apart that your chest can fit between them. Plant your feet directly beneath your knees so you have good, solid support.

Inhale as you lift your arms up over your head. Then exhale as you bend forward from the hips, keeping arms outstretched and keeping your back straight as far as possible. Then, let everything relax and hang down. Let your body hang between your knees and relax.

Take several deep breaths, and every time you exhale be conscious of relaxing a fraction of an inch farther forward.

After several deep breaths, place your hands on top of your knees. Push yourself back up to a sitting position as you inhale.

in the Office

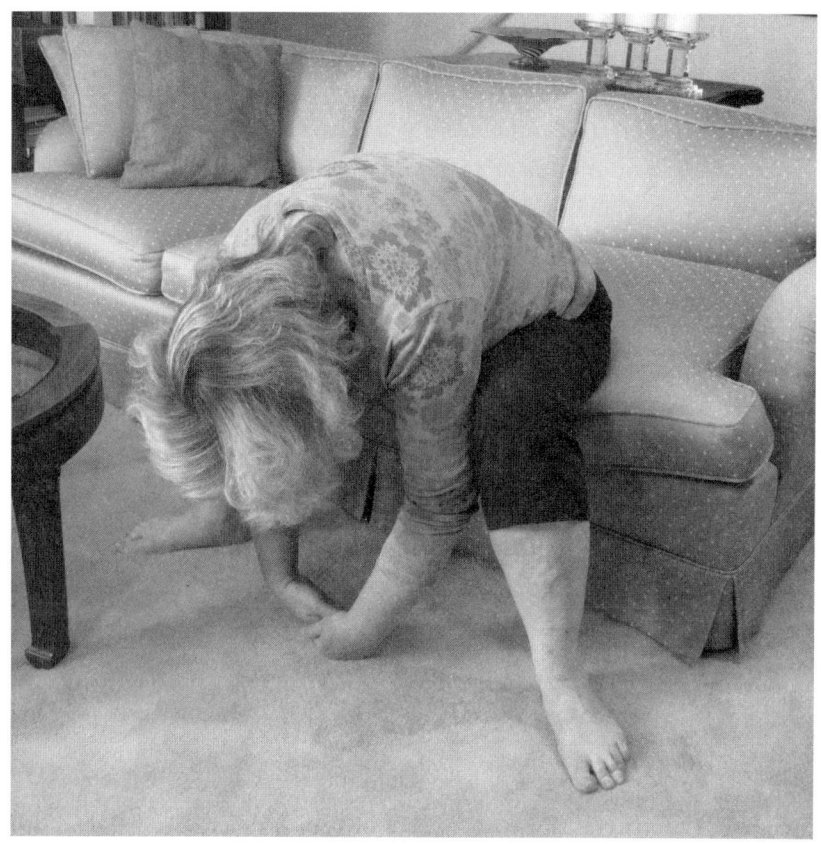

in the Office

Backbend . . . Revisited

After a forward bend, we need to balance the body by bending backwards.

Start sitting on the front edge of your chair. Inhale and lift your chest toward the ceiling. Arch back allowing your arms to rest on the chair seat or sides. Let your head drop back and breathe deeply for several breaths.

Exhale as you sit back up.

You could also do a standing backbend if the seated one won't work for your situation.

in the Office

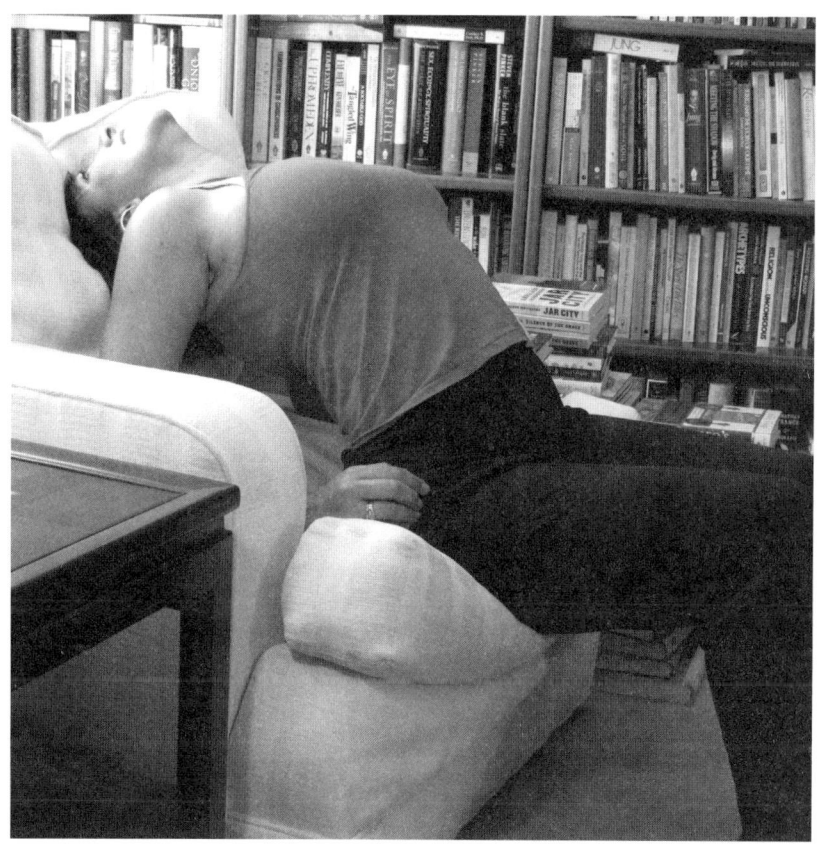

Out of India
You Are a Yogi

The word *yogi* means, "one who practices yoga." That's all. Whether you do daily classes with an instructor, weekly classes with an instructor, or simply the best you can do at home with the time and space you have doesn't matter. If you do yoga to fall asleep, you are a yogi. If you do a kitchen warrior pose while you wait for the cookie timer, you are a yogi.

That being the case, you might like to have some idea of the context into which your practice fits.

Specifically, you are one who practices *hatha* yoga if you follow the practices in this book. Hatha yoga is the physical yoga we in Western culture think of when we hear the word *yoga*. While it is the major form of yoga practiced in the United States, it springs from an immense and varied tradition.

You are the latest in a line of yogis stretching back in time to where history moves from verified to speculation. I've heard it said that the first hatha yoga (physical yoga) arose when meditating hermits found that their bodies just wouldn't stay quiet enough to allow them to meditate as long as they wished to. So they developed the first yoga poses to work the kinks out so they could sit still and contemplate their navels some more. Over millennia (literally), their efforts evolved into the hatha yoga we know.

I love that story. I love the direct connection it makes between the health of the spirit and the health of the body. But if we turn from speculation to what is verifiable, the earliest evidence of yoga comes from an archeological dig in the Indus Valley. They are stone seals showing yogis doing yoga postures. These seals have been dated to around 3000 BCE. So our lineage (yours and mine) goes back 5000 years, give or take a decade or century.

In many spiritual traditions and healing traditions, practitioners talk about their lineage. My shamanic friend talks about his teacher, his teacher's teacher, etc. My Reiki (a hands-on healing technique) teacher can name her lineage back to Reiki's founder. It's difficult for any individual yogi to talk about their personal lineage these days simply because we generally only know the name of our teacher and the "brand" of yoga she or he teaches. But we shouldn't allow lack of knowledge to make us forget that the lineage is there and it is an ancient one.

Hindu/Yoga Scriptural History

The Vedas

The Hindu tradition is blessed with the most ancient religious texts in the world: the Vedas. Written about 4000 years ago, the Vedas are a collection of hymns praising higher power and containing the oldest recorded yoga teachings. They are considered, like the Christian Bible, to be divine revelation. The goal of the yoga teachings in the Vedas is for the yogi to transcend the limitations of the mind.

The Upanishads

About 3500 years ago, writings known as the Upanishads appeared. They explain the relationship between the transcendental self (Atman) and ultimate reality (Brahman). They also introduce the concept of karma. *Historical Note: The Jain religion was born in 1200 BCE and Buddhism in 600 BCE, give or take. Both have roots in Hinduism and yoga tradition.*

The Bhagavad-Gita

The Bhagavad-Gita is the first scripture devoted entirely to yoga. It was written around 2500 years ago (approx. 500 BCE). The Gita, as it is affectionately referred to, is the record of a conversation between Prince Arjuna and Lord Krishna, an avatar of Vishnu, on the battlefield. It is a fascinating moral discussion about karma and morality, and Arjuna's reluctance to kill friends and family members (my interpretation).

The Yoga Sutra

In the second century of our common era, a man named Patanjali wrote the Yoga Sutra in a effort to standardize yoga. I think he may have had obsessive-compulsive disorder to codify everything so precisely. Yet, because he did so, he created a clear thread we can follow back nearly 2000 years. He expounded upon the eightfold path of raja yoga, and the third limb of that eightfold path is the asanas, or poses, of hatha yoga.

Historical Note: The Yoga Sutra has not prevented the proliferation of branches of yoga like hatha yoga and tantric yoga and the many styles of yoga current in the world today. It's more like Patanjali pruned the tree to make it stronger!

Hindu Religion

When I was introduced to yoga philosophy and Hindu religion through my course work in college, I found it to be a satisfying description of reality. I adopted much of it for my own. While what I learned then is indeed the heart and soul of yoga and is inextricably woven through Hindu culture, there is also an almost fundamentalist fervor about how those truths are sometimes passed on. Just as my Christian brother would buttonhole his classmates and ask, "Are you saved?" I've been buttonholed by yogis from India and preached to in New Age stores, at conferences and, once, on the street.

In the West we are told that the Hindu religion is polytheistic because the people worship Vishnu and Indra, Parvati and Kali, Shiva and Shakti—and many others. What is less well known to the Western public is that all of these gods are seen as aspects of one god, the Supreme Being. When people bring offerings to the altar of Ganesha, they know they are petitioning one aspect of God. When I was buttonholed by a yogi, he was not trying to get me to worship the goddess Durga, he was trying to teach me what he knew about the path to Nirvana, or union with God.

Which is, after all, the purpose of yoga in India. The word, *yoga*, means union, or to yoke together, body and mind, mind and spirit, human and god. There is a branch of yoga called raja yoga which is specifically about becoming one with God. There is also a saying, "no raja without hatha, no hatha without raja." Which means, simply, you can't become one with God without being grounded in your body and you can't focus on perfecting your body without being led to union with God.

Of course, the path to union with God through hatha yoga can be a long one if we are only practicing once a week. It's enough to tackle the union of mind and body for most of us. And even in India, raja yoga is not expected of everyone, only those who feel called after a lifetime of meeting one's obligations to society through family and work.

Yoga's Nitty-Gritty

The Eightfold Path

For most of my association with yoga I found the eight limbs of the eightfold path from Patanjali's Yoga Sutra more confusing than useful. They seemed alien and, sometimes, downright weird. I don't know if I will ever be comfortable with the Sanskrit names.

However, when researching for this chapter and being reintroduced to them, I've discovered that I've begun to practice some of them without realizing it. It seems to me now that if we peel away some of the cultural overlays, the eightfold path has gifts to offer those of us practicing yoga in the West.

The eight limbs of yoga are 1) yama, ethical principles, 2) niyama, rules of conduct, 3) asana, postures or the physical exercises of yoga, 4) pranayama, the science of breath, 5) pratyahara, control of the senses, 6) dharana, concentration, 7) dhyana, meditation, and 8) samadhi, union with the divine.

The limbs that are recognized in most hatha yoga practice are asana and pranayama with a little meditation thrown in. It is as though we've surveyed a system meant to work as a whole and just yanked out the parts that made sense to us, leaving valuable parts, unrecognized, behind. This has led to practices that use yoga poses and techniques out of context.

The eight limbs are presented in the order above because each provides a foundation for the next. For instance, the ethical principles expressed in the yamas can be seen as a kind of Hindu Ten Commandments. They list behaviors to avoid and they prepare the yogi for what comes next. Without them we cannot meaningfully practice the niyamas.

Yama

There are five yamas. The first and most familiar to westerners is the one associated with Mahatma Gandhi: **ahimsa** ("You shall not kill," or non-harming). This arises from the recognition that all beings are one with the Supreme Being and as such are part of ourselves. This is why vegetarian eating is fundamental to Hinduism.

I too was a vegetarian for a long time. Not directly because of yoga, but because I loved animals and couldn't bear to harm them. Then I discovered that plants have feelings and spirits as well. My choices became: Become a fruitarian (an extremely expensive way to get enough food to survive on), learn to live on air as certain yogic saints do, or resolve to eat both plants and animals with reverence. That means being gratefully aware of the sacrifices made by other beings for my survival, and making sure that food is prepared in ways that honor the ingredients.

To be alive is to inconvenience other life forms, but also to be of service to them through how we live and what we do with our bodies when we're no longer using them. Ahimsa requires us to take no more than we need and to do what we can for the well-being of our fellow travelers on the planet. Not only other species, but other members of our own species. Christians, Muslims, Hindus, Jews, Buddhists, and Animists have all created beautiful, meaningful ways to make sense of living. Republicans, communists, democrats, sultans, kings and presidents all struggle to make societies work. Sometimes the complexities that societies must accommodate frustrate folks to the point that war or extermination seems the only answer.

Judging others for their beliefs or behaviors does not help. Compassion does. So does holding the ideal of ahimsa in our hearts even when it seems impossible to make it a world-wide reality.

Satya ("You shall not lie"). Mahatma Gandhi said, "Truth is God and God is Truth." My experience with lies demonstrates that they take away bits and pieces of the self and leave you hollow and disconnected. They propel you into living a life of fantasy and take you away from the real beauty of authentic living.

I cannot speak for others, but when I told lies they arose from a fear that who I really am did not measure up to the unknown but all-powerful standard that I thought must exist "out there" somewhere. Through astrology I've come to understand some of the motivation behind the lies that others tell. (jinjerstanton.com/AnatomyLiar) This does not change or diminish the damage that lies do to the teller of them. I could feel my self disintegrating around the edges. It became harder to identify my self. Since I have stopped telling lies I've discovered strength and integrity in my being that I was unaware of before. This convinced me that satya is a very valuable yama that has nothing to do with others and everything to do with the healthy self.

Asteya ("You shall not steal"). Stealing is similar to lying in how it disintegrates the authentic self. We try to differentiate between petty and grand theft just as we believe there is a difference between white lies and the real humdingers. But stealing a dollar is as harmful to our souls as stealing the Mona Lisa would be.

Stealing is part of certain aspects of our culture. Most of us have, at one time or another, been guilty of employee pilferage (paper clips, pens, file folders). It's seen as no big deal. The company can afford it. And most of us have snatched a grape in the grocery store without causing damage to anyone. But it's not harm to others that is the issue here. It is the way these thefts (petty or grand) nibble away at our integrity. Asteya helps us own that which is most valuable to us: our selves.

There is a certain mind-set that says whatever you can get away with is okay. That is only true if you don't value your self. If you don't value your self, existence loses meaning.

Brahmacharya is difficult to translate into Western terms. It literally means "under the tutelage of Brahma." Brahmacharya refers to celibacy, religious study and self-restraint. It resembles expected behavior of monks and nuns in Christian monasteries. Yet in Indian society many people who practice brahmacharya are married with children, because without knowledge of human love one can't know divine love. One way to translate brahmacharya for Western sensibilities may be to see it as cultivating control of all our perception so that we are not unbalanced by our own experience, our hormones, our desires, our fears. This means that we take a step back from the situations we find ourselves in and look at them objectively.

I know from experience how easy it is to take events personally. If a boss yelled at me, I took it personally. If the homeless woman yelled at me because I only had a quarter to give her, I took it personally. If a friend neglected to call, I thought it was because of some fault of mine. The truth is, very few of other people's actions have anything at all to do with me or anything I may have done. That holds true for you as well. Brahmacharya can help us see that.

The other aspect of brahmacharya that intrigues me is the tradition of religious study. The practice of this aspect of brahmacharya has led me to study many metaphysical traditions and opened my eyes to the proverbial "many paths to the one true god."

According to B.K.S. Iyengar, "Brahmacharya is the battery that sparks the torch of wisdom." It is the path to becoming one with God in Hindu tradition. Without it I doubt pratyahara (limb 5) would be possible.

Aparigraha ("You shall not hoard" or "You shall not covet"). Hoarding (or coveting what one doesn't need) shows poverty of spirit and indicates one does not have faith in God. The net result of practicing aparigraha is a life of simplicity with only those things one needs immediately to hand, trusting that when one needs something it will be available. This can be a real challenge in our culture of consumerism.

A colleague of mine, Timothy Cope, illustrated an insidious consequence of hoarding in a recent Sunday service. He talked about a bottle of Worcestershire sauce that he bought to replace an empty one, and how he somehow kept putting off opening the new bottle even though it was his custom to put the sauce on his daily hamburger (can you tell he's a bachelor?). This went on for weeks until he looked at the bottle in the cupboard and asked himself why he was saving it. He owned the condiment, but by not opening it he lost the benefit of having it. I realized I was doing the same with a bottle of expensive maple syrup.

I am also tempted in this direction whenever I come across something old that has a flavor of a by-gone age—even if it isn't to my taste. I feel an odd obligation to hold onto old pottery or the ancient tax returns of someone unrelated to me—for their historical value.

The truth is that holding onto or coveting things (or condiments) of any kind puts a burden on spirit. Even stored neatly away, things clutter life up and obscure its meaning and purpose. Getting rid of excess belongings (as suggested by both spiritual teachers and designers) is literally lightening your load in life.

Niyama

Niyamas are behaviors and ways of being in the world (virtues) that are valuable to cultivate within ourselves. There are five of them just as there are five yamas. They (together with the yamas) provide the fertile bed in which the rest of the limbs can flourish.

Saucha (purity of the body). Saucha incorporates the poses and breathing exercises of hatha yoga with dietary practices and attention to keeping the body clean inside and out. Saucha is considered essential for physical health. In addition, it places great value on mental hygiene and satya (non-lying). Some of the physical cleansing practices are alien and a little scary (like swallowing 15 feet of damp fabric and pulling it out again). Others have been proven to be highly effective in protecting the practitioner from illness (like rinsing the nasal passages with salty water—*see the chapter on Bathroom Yoga*).

Symbolically, when we wash away the dirt of the world, we are washing away worldliness itself and saying we are ready to turn our minds and hearts to something higher. We are showing ourselves to be open to enlightenment, and we feel lighter.

Wiccan ceremonies often begin with a bathing ritual. In Catholic churches congregants dip their hands into holy water before entering. The baptism ceremony in many Christian denominations is all about washing away the past and going forward with a more spiritual consciousness.

Francis Bacon in *Advancement of Learning* (1605) wrote: "Cleanness of body was ever deemed to proceed from a due reverence to God." Yet, though we *say*, "cleanliness is next to godliness" we treat it as part of our secular lives (showering after a workout on the way to work). We have built cleanliness into the mainstream of our culture. We reap the health benefits, but if we were to bring mindfulness to our bathing rituals we might also reap the spiritual benefits.

Santosa (contentment). It's difficult for a person in the midst of stress and striving to be able to meditate or to have his or her mind become "one-pointed." This means that we need some level of contentment in order to practice meditation.

B. K. S. Iyengar, one of the major teachers who brought yoga to the United States, says, "A contented man is . . . blessed because he has known truth and joy." To "know truth and joy" we need to *stop*. We need to be still and present to what's happening *right now*. We need to see that the sunset tonight has its own glory and the breeze right now carries its own unique perfume.

To develop a sense of contentment, try keeping a gratitude journal in which you write down, every day, five things you are grateful for (as seen on Oprah, for one). Or rewrite your life story in terms of lessons learned, blessings received and successes earned. Read it every day instead of telling yourself and others the hard luck story of your life. I promise you, there is more good in most people's lives than they ever realize. Concentrating on the good in yours can transform it!

Tapas (to burn/commitment/consistency). This niyama is not described consistently in the literature and is very difficult to get a handle on. Many descriptions make it sound like a kind of religious fervor, something familiar to Christianity and Islam as well.

Yet, the translation "to burn" seems to indicate a burning away of whatever prevents us from expressing our truest selves or distracts us from a clear focus on our personal goals (either imposed from outside or from within). It may seem paradoxical to set tapas beside santosa (contentment). Yet the burning away of irrelevancies in our lives can leave space for contentment to develop.

"To burn" also points toward passion for self-expression which is closely related to living with integrity and following your own internal guidance. Tapas means making those things that feed our souls (yoga or music, nature or cooking) a priority in life at least on a par with work, paying taxes or getting the kids to soccer practice. It means passion for what feeds us, and lovingly tending our internal flame.

Svadhyaya (study). This one has both inner and outer components. It means both self-study and self-education. In yoga tradition it is taken to mean study of God and the study of God within the individual. Many assume this indicates a very narrow scope of study. That's not necessarily true.

To me it means exploring my own nature—getting to know who I really am. Since I am not only this body and this personality, it means learning about the universe around me, studying both philosophy and physics, as well as learning how to sail or play a sousaphone. It also means learning about the people in the world around me because we are all connected and what I learn about them, I learn about myself as well. All things reflect the nature of god or the divine. By studying all of this my quality of life improves and my understanding of the divine increases. This is true for any aspect of life I was unfamiliar with before.

And if science is your religion? Studies have shown that people who make a priority of continual learning have a better quality of life as they age. New neural pathways are continually being created, which keeps the brain flexible and protects it from deterioration.

Isvara Pranidhana (surrender to God). I've seen it translated "dedication to God" or dedicating one's actions to God. This is a big virtue in Christianity too. But Buddhism, which isn't known for devotion to a god, promotes this virtue as well. Buddhists call the concept *non-attachment*. It arises from one of the Buddha's *Four Noble Truths:* "All suffering arises from desire." Desire leads to attachment. A great line I found on beliefnet.com is, "By holding onto that which in any case is forever slipping through our fingers, we just get rope burn."

But if we do what must be done, or what is at hand to do, and we let go of the outcome, we take ourselves outside the cycle of suffering. If we do the best that is within our power and turn the rest over to "God," we let go of huge burdens. We can be happy whatever the outcome of our efforts.

That letting go of outcomes is one of the tougher disciplines. It is also very powerful. Worrying about outcomes keeps us from enjoying the here and now and also, sometimes, from doing the best we can right now or taking advantage of opportunities.

Problems arise when we as individuals think God wants infidels dead and the sinful to be punished. I say, if that's what God wants, let God take care of it. I'll do the best I can here and now and strive not to be attached to what other people do or don't do. I feel happier already.

Asana

We in the West tend to practice the *asanas,* or postures/exercises for purely physical reasons. We want to become stronger, more flexible, healthier and stay physically young. The postures help our bodies move through life more easily. I have seen my own students grow younger by practicing yoga. There are plenty of physical disciplines that provide some (though seldom all) of the same physical benefits. But asana, practiced with spiritual intent, brings the mind to the present moment and a fine awareness of the interplay of mind and body. It reveals to us the way mind and body interact with spirit. Asana grounds us in the here and now as a kind of mindfulness meditation.

Pranayama

The word *prana* in Sanskrit means both breath and spirit. In English, the word *respiration* comes from the same root as the word spirit. I've often wondered how widespread in the world's languages the connection between breath and spirit is. There is a level at which yogic tradition sees the two as literally the same. *Ayama* means control; therefore, *pranayama* is breath control, and it leads to greater awareness of spirit. B. K. S. Iyengar describes pranayama as "the hub around which the wheel of life revolves." Cultivation of breath control, even just bringing attention to the breath, is a useful first step toward a meditation practice.

There are a variety of breathing exercises used by yogis, but it's vital to learn how to breathe properly first. (*See* To Breathe Properly *in "Yoga Basics" on page 4*.) Once a deep, slow, rhythmic breath becomes habit is soon enough to look into the more advanced breathing techniques.

Pratyahara

Pratyahara is "removing the tentacles of consciousness from the world." We detach our attention from the world outside of us: people, situations, sensations, things, yesterday and tomorrow. We also let go of our thoughts about these externals. Pranayama is a great first step. By concentrating on your breath to the exclusion of all else you have already begun the practice of pratyahara. If you've ever become so totally absorbed in a task or project that you lost all track of time or consciousness of activity happening around you, you've experienced something very like pratyahara. The next step is to let go of your task or project or the process of breathing.

Pratyahara is considered a sort of linchpin in the pursuit of union with the divine, a vital step toward disentangling yourself from the world of illusion. It is also a bridge to meditation in the final three limbs of yoga.

Dharana

One way to look at *dharana* is to reach out to the divine with the tentacles you just removed from the world. The idea is to concentrate all of our attention on the infinite. The difficulty with that is that we may not understand what it means to reach out in this way. Try using the word AUM (often written as OM) as a focus of concentration because it stands for the Creator who transcends the limitations of time (A: the beginning, U: the middle, M: completion). Dharana is the first step in meditation.

Dhyana

Dhyana is the second step of meditation. At this stage the effort involved in focusing our consciousness dissolves and we are conscious only of our own existence and the existence of the object of meditation. This state is often described as "bliss" and it is not something we can just choose to "do." It comes unbidden when we are "doing" other things like pranayama, pratyahara or dharana.

Samadhi

Contact with God is the goal of all eight limbs of yoga and the state of union with God is *samadhi*. It is the final step in meditation where the consciousness of being separate from the divine dissolves. Both this and *dhyana* can occur unexpectedly when one is practicing dharana without expectation. Until that happens they can seem mythological. One need not be Hindu or practicing yoga to experience samadhi. We can be transported into union with the divine without seeking it. It comes to us most often in nature when we are awed by the mountains, the sea or the opening of a flower.

The Value of Meditation

In our daily lives, the goal of union with the divine may seem impractical, even impossible, and dedicating time to the practice of meditation can even seem selfish. Yet meditation has very real and measurable benefits for our everyday life. Meditators experience less stress and fewer of the health problems associated with it. Meditation helps us respond to events in our lives in a more healthy manner and even to enjoy life more, because we are more present in the moment rather than worrying about the past or future. A less well-known benefit of meditation is that the people around meditators experience benefits too. The calm is catching. Business meetings become more productive and family disagreements less volatile without effort. A study took place in India (mentioned by Deepak Chopra in one of his books) that showed that if just one percent of the populations meditates, violence in that area decreases significantly.

Dharana, dhyana and samadhi offer us a path to greater wholeness, and perhaps a deeper connection to our own souls and a more peaceful world. It can begin with something as simple as paying attention to the breath.

Other Useful Things to Know About

The Energetic Body

The energetic body is recognized in many ancient healing traditions including Cherokee, Chinese, and Hindu. In Hindu or Ayurvedic tradition there are vortices of energy called "chakras." The word *chakra* in Sanskrit means wheel or disk. While there are many chakras located throughout the body, most people in the West who use the word are referring to the seven major chakras that are located along the spine and in the head.

The condition of these chakras has repercussions not only for physical health but for the very shape a person's life takes. For instance, a weak root chakra can be seen in a person's life through struggles with money and the basics of staying alive. A healthy root chakra would be seen in the relative stability of a person's life and a lack of worry around financial or survival issues.

The root chakra is also referred to as the first chakra and is located at the very base of the spine.

The second chakra (sacral) is located a couple of inches below the navel and pertains to sex, passion and generative creativity.

Chakra three (solar plexus) is about two inches above the navel and has to do with a person's ability to attain his or her goals. It also has to do with personal power.

The bridge between the lower chakras and the higher chakras is the fourth or heart chakra (guess where it's located). Predictably it has to do with love and compassion.

Number five is the chakra located at the base of the throat. It is literally our ability to express ourselves through words, to speak our truth.

In the center of the forehead just between the eyebrows is the sixth chakra (third eye) which is the center of our ability to "see" both literally and metaphorically. It is also our doorway to "second sight."

Finally, the seventh chakra (crown) which is located at the very top of the skull is our connection to the infinite, the divine.

Connecting these and the other chakras of the body are the nadis or lines of energy in the body. They roughly correspond to the meridians of traditional Chinese medicine.

Tools and Practices

Mudras: Nadis run down through the fingers, and by positioning the fingers in certain ways you can affect how the energy flows. The various finger positions are called mudras. The most famous mudra is the Guyan mudra where the tips of the index finger and thumb meet. It's very popular for sitting meditation. You can think of mudras as yoga for the fingers.

Mudras are found around the world. Jesus is often shown with his hands in mudras. Placing the hands together in the prayer position is using a mudra. The European "sign against the evil eye" is a mudra. Even in the ancient carvings of pre-Columbian America mudras are portrayed.

Mantras: One means of focusing the mind for meditation is the use of mantras. A mantra is a word or phrase repeated either verbally or mentally. Aum is most common (often shortened to Om). According to Iyengar, Aum and the Latin "omni" come from the same root meaning "all." Aum represents divinity and the infinite, so it makes a great mantra for meditation.

Mandalas and Yantras: Mandalas and yantras are also a focus for meditation. In Hindu tradition they are usually geometric images made up of triangles, squares, circles and lotus blossoms with varying numbers of petals. The terms seem to be used interchangeably; however, most often yantra is used in Hindu contexts and is more geometric. Mandala is generally used in Buddhist contexts and is more pictorial. I have not been able to verify this, but I heard that experiments were done with chanting Aum over a layer of very fine sand on a thin membrane. The pattern the vibration created in the sand was identical to the yantra connected with the mantra Aum. Hmmm . . .

A Sampling of Yoga Styles

Ancient as the traditions are, yoga itself is a living, breathing entity that evolves and changes as the needs of yogis change. Today it takes a myriad forms depending on how the attitudes, life-styles and physical predilections of human beings change. Below are just a sampling of yoga flavors. When choosing for yourself, choose a teacher who speaks in a way that makes sense to you, and a style of yoga that harmonizes with your personal situation. I, for instance, would faint if I practiced Bikram Yoga! Also, keep in mind that even if a class is called Iyengar or Ashtanga it may not bear much similarity to what its originator had in mind. Most yoga in the United States is some form of hatha yoga and I'll only talk below about hatha yoga types.

Ananda Yoga: Legacy of Paramahansa Yogananda

Paramahansa Yogananda's book, *Autobiography of a Yogi* inspired me. I'm not alone. Out of his teachings arose the Self-Realization Fellowship, *Ananda Yoga* (developed by his disciple, Swami Kriyananda). Ananda yoga is a classical style of hatha yoga that focuses on awakening and controlling the subtle energies within. In this style of yoga you would hear far more about chakras than in most styles. It is one of the gentler forms of yoga with a more internal focus.

Anusara Yoga

Anusara (a-nu-SAR-a) means "to move with the current of divine will." A new style developed by John Friend, Anusara Yoga is described as spiritually inspiring, yet grounded in a deep knowledge of how the body works. The abilities and limitations of each individual student is honored. If a yoga style can be said to have a motto, Anusara's would be, "attitude, action and alignment."

Ashtanga Yoga

In the United States Ashtanga Yoga is associated with Pattabhi Jois. It is physically demanding and best for those who want a serious workout. Participants jump from one pose to the next with no breaks. Many celebrities are Ashtanga yogis. It's great for building strength and stamina. Vinyasa is a variety of Ashtanga Yoga. Power yoga is based on Ashtanga.

Bikram Yoga

Bikram Yoga is named for Bikram Choudhury, its founder, who studied with Paramahansa Yogananda's brother. Bikram Yoga is practiced in a room heated up to 100 degrees and consists of a series of 26 asanas. Each posture is usually performed twice and held for a certain period of time. The theory is that the body is more flexible at the high temperatures. Maybe, but I wouldn't be conscious to find out. People who are cold all the time normally love Bikram. It is supposed to aid the body in releasing toxins, and I see how that would be. Don't start this kind of yoga unless you are already in top shape. It also is popular with celebs.

Iyengar Yoga

This style of yoga was founded by B. K. S. Iyengar who believed that "in each pose there should be repose." The focus is on precise alignment, which is why Iyengar Yoga is known for its uses of props (straps and blocks) to make it easier to achieve the postures. While a beginner can take these classes, feedback from those who have suggests that the beginner should be fit to begin with. It can be strenuous.

Kripalu Yoga

Kripalu Yoga was developed by Amrit Desai, a yogi from India. He founded the Kripalu Center in Lenox, Massachusetts. This is a mindful yoga style with an emphasis on listening to the body as the poses are performed. The individual student is encouraged to listen to his or her own body wisdom while doing the poses. This is the style closest to what I practice myself.

Kundalini Yoga

While the focus of this style of yoga is the controlled release of the kundalini (or "serpent") energy, usually visualized as a snake coiled at the base of the spine, it incorporates asana, meditation and pranayama as the tools to achieve that goal. As the Kundalini awakens, it moves up through all of the chakras to the crown chakra. At that point one achieves samadhi. More tangible benefits are increased health and vitality.

Svaroopa Yoga

Svaroopa Yoga (which is becoming more common) focuses on "core opening" to lift pressure off your internal organs and glands. Stress relief and deep relaxation are some of the benefits. It uses blankets folded in creative ways to support the body for the desired position. This is not for people looking for a strenuous workout.

Resources

This is the smallest representation of the resources available for pursuing your interest in yoga. A mere jumping off place.

BOOKS

These are grouped according to ease in terms of physical challenge presented. It happens that as the physical difficulty increases, so does the weight of the theory and philosophy! This is a small selection with a wide range of appeal.

Babar's Yoga for Elephants

Laurent de Brunhoff, Harry N. Abrams, 2002
A nice bit of nostalgia for those who loved Babar as children. I don't know how inspired children might be with it (or whether they would even be able to do all the poses) but as a basic reference of poses with clear illustrations for adults it is nice (just remember to use a belt when the elephant recommends a trunk). One good thing is you can lay the book open flat (the hard cover at least).

The Little Yoga Book

Erika Dillman, Warner Books, 1999
A 6-by-6-inch gem that contains the moving personal story of the authors healing through yoga as well as wonderful sketches of the poses.

It also has nice descriptions of the benefits of the poses and how to do them. If you want to know the Sanskrit names of the poses, it provides them as well.

The New Yoga for People Over 50

Suza Francina, Health Communications, 1997

The students in my yoga classes represent a wide range of ages, and even the younger people need to start off with easier versions of some poses. This book addresses many of the issues older beginners may have, like arthritis, menopause and heart health. It is friendly and accessible as well as chock-full of information. It recommends specific exercises for specific physical challenges as well as offering options for using props to make some of the poses easier to attain and maintain.

Yoga, Youth and Reincarnation

Jess Stearn, Doubleday, 1963

This book was written by professional skeptic, Jess Stearn. He wrote books on psychic ability, Edgar Cayce and reincarnation. He told stories in journalistic style about subjects rejected by the mainstream society of his time. He was one of us, whoever you consider "us" to be. In this book he shares some fantastic tales about his yoga teacher (Marcia Moore, who went on to become a controversial figure in the exploration of altered consciousness), his own experience of yoga and some practical information that can help us practice yoga. It includes a fine set of asanas to help the newcomer get started.

Light on Yoga

B. K. S. Iyengar, Schocken Books, 1966

Iyengar is the founder of one of the major schools of yoga in the United States. It is a demanding and strenuous variety of yoga that stresses the use of props to aid in achieving perfect alignment. This book is crammed full of photos of poses that can scare some people away from yoga. It also contains a good discription of the finer points of yoga tradition. But, unless you are remarkably flexible and strong already, look at the poses illustrated as examples of human potential or as entertainment, at least until you have built up your own strength and flexibility.

The Complete Illustrated Book of Yoga

Swami Vishnudevananda, Julian Press, 1960

Again, illustrations should be taken as potential, not as expectation. The primary value of this book to me is the discussion of some of the yogic practices often seen by Westerners as bizarre. Admittedly, some of them I cannot envision ever trying—even if future studies prove their worth. Others, such as tongue cleaning and rinsing the nose with salty water *(see Bathroom Yoga: Neti Pot)* have been proven to have real value in maintaining health and are worth practicing. I also have come to value the gazing exercises, but remember to not push yourself beyond your own comfort. The swami suggests starting with minute-long sessions. I suggest starting with a few seconds at a time.

MAGAZINES

Yoga Journal

Bi-Monthly Magazine
My old friend. As I've grown over the years, so has *Yoga Journal*. It makes a real effort to be accurate and to cover all aspects of yoga in the U.S. and the world. Great articles about individual poses, what their benefits are, and how to work toward the more difficult ones. Also, thoughtful articles about the philosophy of yoga and how it applies to modern life along with interviews with important figures in the world of yoga. That's just the tip of the iceberg. The information can be extremely dense. I keep old issues for reference.

Fit Yoga

You could think of this as yoga light, but not lite. It takes yoga seriously, but light-heartedly. The information is less dense and sometimes more basic than *Yoga Journal* without talking down to beginners. I like the clear illustrations and the friendly editorial slant. Very approachable while being informative.

Yoga International

Himalayan Institute
This magazine has its roots planted firmly in Mother India via the Himalayan Institute.

Hinduism Today

Kauai's Hindu Monastery
If you are interested in Hinduism, I recommend *Hinduism Today Magazine*. Published quarterly from Kauai's Hindu Monastery, it is the foremost global journal on Hinduism. It is sensible and provides a broad perspective on the many faces of Hinduism without coming from an alien perspective. It is aimed at practicing Hindus, so it is not about converting outsiders.

VIDEO/DVD

I have sampled videos and DVDs looking particularly at those aimed at beginners. If you are not sure about any of these, take them out of a library to try them before buying so that if following along is too frustrating you won't have the video or DVD on your shelf mocking you. Remember to listen to your own body and to be gentle with yourself as you work through any recording.

Living Arts and/or Yoga Journal Videos

Featuring Rodney Yee or Patricia Walden
Nice production values and good information, but beginners who are not already fit and flexible will find some of the transitions very difficult, and will only be able to approximate some of the poses shown. *AM Yoga for Beginners* and *Yoga Journal's Practice for Relaxation* seem accessible to most. While they mention props at the beginning of each video they seldom show their use.

Yoga Zone Videos

There are some inspirational aspects to these videos. The demonstrators are of diverse body shapes and in the Yoga for Weight Loss video they show one person doing easier versions of the poses and another doing the traditional pose. They also show possible pitfalls we could fall into. They are encouraging, and conscious that not all viewers will be able to do everything right away.

WEBSITES

Oh, the sites that are available! Here are three reliable starting points.

Yoga Journal

http://www.yogajournal.com

The *Yoga Journal* website takes the magazine's content to a whole new level. It contains an enormous backlog of past articles about all aspects of yoga. Related articles are cross-referenced with one another so that if you are reading an article about how to do an inverted pose, you can easily shift to an article about the benefits of inversions. There is also a substantial library about many other aspects of yoga like philosophy, diet and leaders in the yoga community. This is a fantastic resource for going deeper into Western yoga.

ABC of Yoga

http://www.abc-of-yoga.com/default.asp
I like the straight-forward, no-nonsense approach of this site. It is about basics. The different pages of the site are laid out to one side like the chapters of a book, with free information at the top and shopping opportunities toward the bottom. The basic information in this site can be accessed easily and directly leaving you with a decent overview of yoga, the styles of yoga and most basic poses. It is not a deep site but it is useful.

And, my personal favorite:

Jinjer Stanton

http://www.jinjerstanton.com
Find back issues of my newsletter here and additional articles about yoga—and other things. To receive my newsletter email me at jinjer@usiwireless.com with the word *newsletter* in the subject line.

Namaste,

    or "the spirit in me salutes the spirit in you."
    We're all in bodies together.

                                      Jinjer

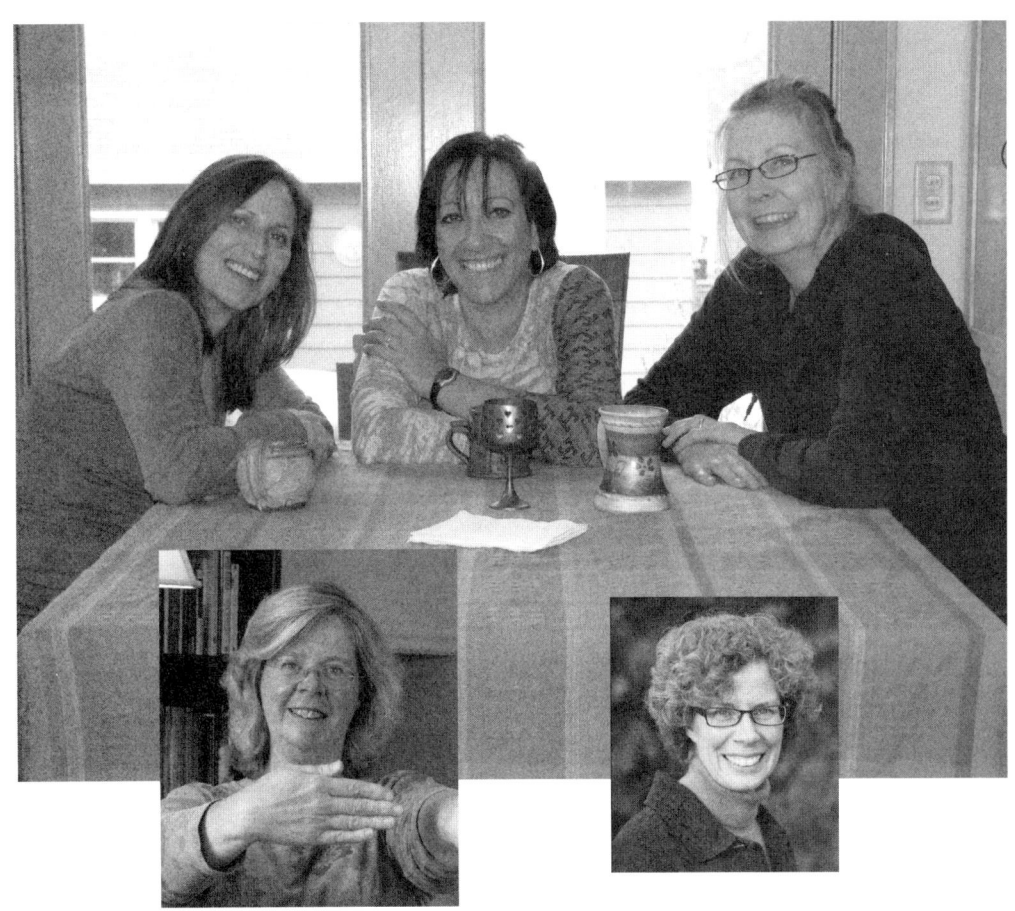

Our models: Cherie Olausen, Yvonne Peralta, Roseann Mammoser, inserts: Susan Olsen, Marcia Thomas

Acknowledgments

This book is not the result of my efforts alone. Indeed there would not be a book were it not for the inspiration and support of many people. Some of them are mentioned here. I want to thank:

Carol Singer who generated the first sliver of the idea and has been untiring in her willingness to proofread again and again.

Myra Duncan who forced me to consider alternative ways to do poses when there are fewer limbs than most people expect.

All of the students I've had over the years for the lessons they've taught me!

I feel honored that these students generously became my models in this book: Susan Olsen, Cherie Olausen, Roseann Mammoser, Yvonne Peralta and Marcia Thomas.

Thank you all from the bottom of my heart.

Others have contributed along the way: friends, colleagues and agents. Thank you all as well.

         Namaste,
         Jinjer

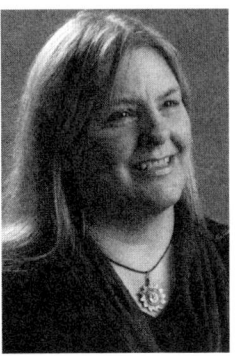

Jinjer Stanton

lives in Minneapolis, Minnesota, where she's been teaching yoga more than ten years. She also gardens, cooks, and rides her bike in the city's beautiful parks.